Muscle Beach

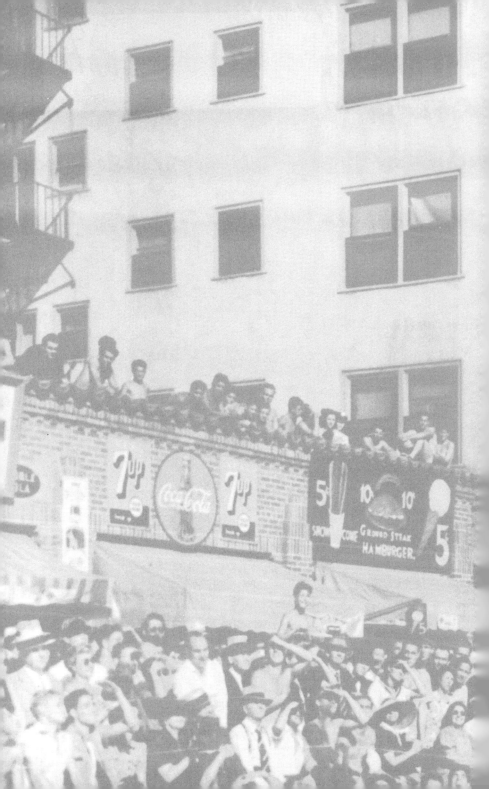

Muscle
Beach

Marla Matzer Rose

AN LA WEEKLY BOOK
FOR ST. MARTIN'S GRIFFIN
NEW YORK

LA Weekly Books is a trademark of LA Weekly Media, Inc.

Cover photo (also on text page 48): George Eiferman and Mim Sharlock on the sand near the platform. Courtesy George Eiferman.

Title page photo spread: A holiday weekend crowd circa 1939: Deforest "Moe" Most with Bruce Conner on his shoulders and an unidentified man on top. Part of this photo also appears on the first page of each chapter.

Photos on pages ii, iii, 11, 17, 20, 28, 31, 40, 42, 44, 47, 51, 57, 59, 60, 63, 69, 87, 89, 119, 131, 147, 149, 159 are from the collection of Les and Pudgy Stockton.

Photos on pages 48, 77, and 78 courtesy of George Eiferman.

BOOK DESIGN BY CASEY HAMPTON

ISBN 0-312-24539-4

First Edition: March 2001

10 9 8 7 6 5 4 3 2 1

For Andy

Contents

Preface

I'd lived in Santa Monica—a city about twenty miles west of downtown Los Angeles, on the Pacific Ocean—for more than three years before I became aware that the "original" Muscle Beach had existed there from the 1930s through the 1950s. As far as I knew, the place in Venice they called Muscle Beach, which I'd passed by a couple of times, was the one and only.

I first heard about Santa Monica's Muscle Beach from a friend who worked out with a couple of bodybuilders. In conversation, they brought up Santa Monica's bodybuilding days. It seemed, the friend reported, that the place that had preceded Venice's Muscle Beach had been closed down in the wake of a sex scandal in the late 1950s.

Bodybuilders in the 1950s? Sex scandals? I was intrigued by the story of the first Muscle Beach. As a frequenter of "muscle" gyms myself (in a very noncompetitive sort of way), and as a student of pop culture and American studies, I was fascinated by the place's history.

The amount of relatively recent yet little-known history in

L.A. has always amazed me—and frustrated me, since I believe Los Angeles has a wealth of recent history that others, particularly New York media types, don't give it credit for, although I was pleased by the attention such publications as the *New York Times* gave to Steve Reeves's obituary in 2000. Back in 1991, I contacted several people about my desire to write a short article on Muscle Beach past and present for *California* magazine, the successor to *New West*, where I then worked.

I was directed by a parks and recreation department employee to Steve Ford, an amateur bodybuilder and a volunteer publicist for Muscle Beach. Ford ended up putting me in touch with most of the people I've relied on as sources for this book.

At the time, Ford told me all that remained of the first Muscle Beach was a small plaque, welded to a tall pole in the sand at the original location just south of the Santa Monica Pier. It replaced an earlier plaque nailed to a shorter pole, which was promptly stolen. It was a first step toward recognition, and perhaps a return of sorts, of Muscle Beach at its original site.

On my first trip to see the plaque, I stopped by the Santa Monica visitors' information booth not far from the pier. There, I inquired about the location of Muscle Beach. The blue-haired lady inside the booth screwed up her face and replied sourly: "Muscle Beach is closed."

Eventually, I learned why, three decades later, some of the older citizens of Santa Monica still bore animosity toward a place that brought so many people joy, and the city so much notoriety. I also came to understand why the history of Muscle Beach isn't more widely known, even in its own backyard.

It's a complicated, sometimes messy, and often contentious subject. It's not just about sport, but about sociology, politics, and business. It doesn't fit neatly into the confines of a single subject, and even the year that Muscle Beach got its start is the subject of some debate among those who were there in the early days.

I hope to give a sense of where Muscle Beach fit into the culture of the time, and how it affected fitness and entertainment today. I've made every effort to make this an accurate, but not a strictly scholarly, volume. I have personally interviewed about a dozen people who were there in the early days of Muscle Beach. I've also used accounts written by other Muscle Beach alumni within the last twelve years, and referred to contemporaneous articles from the press during Muscle Beach's heyday.

There are some excellent recent works that fill the scholarly niche, for those who want to delve deeper into history or into particular areas of interest. Harvey Green's *Fit for America* and John D. Fair's *Muscletown USA* are both fine books on the history of fitness, written by history professors. *Muscletown* in particular presents some fascinating background for the story of Muscle Beach, since its subject, publisher and York Barbell founder Bob Hoffman, was a major force behind the mid-century boom in weight lifting.

The newsletter *Iron Game History* is another interesting resource for scholarly articles on fitness history. It is published by iron game (weight lifting, power lifting, and bodybuilding) enthusiasts/historians Jan and Terry Todd of the University of Texas at Austin.

—Marla Matzer Rose
Los Angeles, California
November 2000

Acknowledgments

Although this book contains both, I never envisioned this as a pure oral or pictorial history of the beach. That is the realm of the Muscle Beach Alumni Association, and several of its members (including Steve Ford), who have collected the stories of Santa Monica's Muscle Beachers and have already turned them into books of their own, or have plans to. I wish them all well; there will always be another story, another perspective, to be told. Though I did not set out to record oral histories, my most treasured and inspiring sources were the people who were there at Muscle Beach in the early days. Most have stayed active in the world of fitness as it has evolved. These individuals provided not only a historical perspective but a fuller understanding of Muscle Beach's impact on today's immense fitness culture as well. First and foremost, I need to thank Les and Abbye "Pudgy" Stockton, perhaps Muscle Beach's most-famous, still-together couple, for their great help and support.

Also generous with their time and recollections were Armand Tanny, George Eiferman, and Gypsy Boots. At least half a dozen other people from the original Muscle Beach also contributed to my research over the course of writing this book. I thank all of them.

Joe Jares, son of the late weight lifter and wrestler Frank Jares and an accomplished sportswriter in his own right, was helpful. He directed me to the Amateur Athletic Foundation's Paul Ziffren Sports Resource Center in Los Angeles, a useful trove of information. Finally, special thanks go to Scott Kaufer for helping me get to the next step as a writer; to Peter McAlevey, who interested me in doing my first magazine story on Muscle Beach; and to Steve Ford, who gave me the key to unlock that which shouldn't be kept secret.

Muscle Beach

The Foundations of the Modern Fitness Movement

Fitness in America didn't start at Muscle Beach. Although the plaque that now stands at the original site of Muscle Beach proclaims it "The Birthplace of the Physical Fitness Boom of the Twentieth Century," the place didn't spring up or exist in a vacuum.

The Greeks and Romans, of course, provided the original model on which the tenets of the modern fitness movement have been based. The concept of the gymnasium, of progressive weight training, and of competitions such as the Olympics were all born in ancient Greece.

Organized exercise was one of the many casualties of the fall of the Roman Empire. Fitness as we know it today in the West was largely forgotten from that time until the Renaissance, when several authors began writing again of weight training and gymnastic exercises. The movement grew very slowly until the nineteenth century, when a number of factors conspired to start bringing the idea of exercise to the general public once more.

By the mid-1800s, the practice of gymnastics and the use of

Indian clubs—weighted wooden clubs that looked somewhat like bowling pins—had gained some popularity as exercise methods. The use of Indian clubs, like most of the exercise forms that would come to sweep across Europe and the United States, was "discovered" by Europeans, who then evangelized them to the rest of the Western world. The story goes that British military men stationed in India in the mid-1800s found that Indian soldiers built muscle through the use of weighted wooden clubs. They adapted the use of these clubs and brought the practice back to England.

From there, it spread to Continental Europe and to America through the efforts of health reformers, publications, and businessmen eager to cash in on the growing interest in fitness. Because the clubs' size could be tailored to any body and because their use was an activity that could be done with little equipment, Indian clubs became popular with women as well as men. By the 1880s, church ladies around America had formed "swing clubs," which met regularly to exercise with Indian clubs.

American women had been encouraged to practice fitness since midcentury. Health reformers like Catherine Beecher—sister of author Harriet Beecher Stowe—were preaching the benefits of healthful, "simple" foods and exercise by mid-century. Beecher was a particularly strong advocate of a healthful diet and exercise for females, and she wrote illustrated books on fitness for girls.

As for weight training, companies were beginning to sell barbells, long metal poles with adjustable weights on each end, by the turn of the century. These were direct precursors of the "modern," plate-loading barbell that was introduced in Germany in the late 1920s and became the model for virtually all barbells today.

Throughout the nineteenth century, there were many promoters of the cause of health and fitness, as America started to shift to an industrial economy and people increasingly led sedentary lives. The cause became somewhat connected to the Progressive movement in the early 1900s, especially with sickly-child-turned-robust-outdoorsman Teddy Roosevelt at the helm of the country. In 1904 Roosevelt was pictured in "Rough Rider"–style garb on the cover of *Physical Culture,* the leading fitness magazine in America for several decades.

The whole concept of leisure and the idea of having to maintain one's health became much more of an issue with the advent of the industrial economy. In an agrarian nation, one was tied to the land and the cycles of nature. It was unthinkable to take time off for a holiday in peak season, and the work itself kept people healthy: they were outdoors, active, eating fresh foods. Once workers moved indoors, into factories and offices, that all changed.

Probably the single most popular and influential piece of fitness apparatus ever introduced in the United States took hold in the late 1800s: the bicycle. There had been precursors to the bicycle for several decades, with large front wheels and no brakes. But the introduction of the modern bike and its mass production in the 1890s was a huge breakthrough. Both men and women took to cycling for transportation, health, and enjoyment.

The surge of interest in health and fitness in nineteenth-century America was also linked to the classical revival that had already swept the arts. Prussian-born Eugen Sandow, an extremely popular strongman of his day who is now largely forgotten, achieved international fame at the Chicago World's Fair of 1893, posing as a classical Greek statue.

To complete the effect, Sandow covered his nearly nude body in white powder. Americans began to appreciate the human form as depicted in classical art, and to ask themselves why they couldn't look like that themselves. Sandow and others capitalized on this, marketing scores of exercise systems and dietary supplements of varying effectiveness. The use of famous strongman Sandow's name on various "health" products became the blueprint for today's health entrepreneurs, who often license their names to diet supplements, exercise equipment, apparel, and the like.

Some nineteenth-century health crusades had more than a grain of truth to them. The basic principles advocated by people like Beecher remain sound today: simple foods in moderate quantities, along with regular exercise. Others advocated regimens that would be considered more than a little nutty today. Scores of worthless "treatments" and patent medicines were sold in the name of health. Some would say things haven't changed much since then.

But at least on a small scale, modern fitness ideals were beginning to take hold as far back as the mid-nineteenth century. The Young Men's Christian Association transformed itself into an organization dedicated to sports and fitness, promoting the idea of "muscular Christianity." According to Harvey Green in *Fit for America,* there were at least seven independent gymnasiums in New York City by 1860.

The rise of these gyms filled with exercise equipment, though hardly modern by today's standards, was significant. Exercise was promoted as a way to cure a variety of ailments as well as to produce a more attractive body.

This new attitude toward exercise signified a move away from simply taking "cures" in pill or liquid form as a way to produce desirable traits such as stamina, or combat undesirable ones such as lethargy. Instead, the message of the modern fitness movement was that it was both possible and desirable to positively affect one's health and reshape one's body through exercise.

This philosophy was one of the hallmarks of the Americanized fitness movement, versus its European roots. The Europeans seemed to be more able to accept exercise and physicality for its own sake. Whether it was the Europeans' greater affinity for ancient cultures or their freedom from an overriding puritanical view of the world, they didn't seem to have as much need to "excuse" the act of developing the body.

Americans, by contrast, seemed to need to justify taking an active interest in their bodies; attaching a belief of a "greater good" to exercise helped them to not feel guilty about it. A century later and much removed in philosophy, America of the twentieth century was ideally poised to make media stars out of its athletes. Thus, not just the physical bigness but the size of their fame came to distinguish American muscle athletes from their European counterparts in time.

Making stars of musclemen also played into the selling of fitness to the masses. Like any effective sales pitch, the case for getting fit was best made by appealing to the psychological and emotional factors behind the desire for fitness, strength, and increased muscle mass.

Premier salesmen like Charles Atlas played on the fear of humiliation: don't get sand kicked in your face, get big and muscular. Much later, in the days of coed workouts, many gyms encouraged the image of their clubs as "pickup" spots. For many, this was a much more attractive motivation to exercise than the mere idea of exercising because it's good for you.

Most of us connect with fitness because we want to look good and we think it will make us look better. People react to the way other people look: we both admire and fear large men, we celebrate and desire beautiful, toned women. The widespread use of cosmetic surgery has upped the ante yet again, but the fact remains that virtually anyone can look better through fitness training. When teamed with a promise of increased health and extended life span, the lure of greater sex appeal (and sexual prowess) is enough to get millions of us to join gyms.

It can also be argued that we've come so far today as to view our bodies as the ultimate wardrobe basic. The fashion trend in the last couple of decades, particularly in women's clothing, has been toward formfitting, rather simple, and even plain clothes that show off a good body rather than decorating or concealing it. Clothing is just a wrapper for the toned form underneath.

This is particularly true among the most looks-conscious element: film and television celebrities whose livelihoods depend on physical appearance. Fashion critics who decry the "death of glamour" today are missing the point: like it or not, the new, dressed-down styles say the person wearing them has nothing to prove and nothing to hide. Her slim, toned body alone is evidence of her power; she has the knowledge, the time, and the money to achieve that sought-after look.

A few words about the terms used in this book to describe various forms of exercise: there are certain terms, such as *weight lifting,* that have a specific meaning to athletes. Whereas "lifting weights" can mean any form of exercise that employs the use of weights in resistance training, "weight lifting" in the strict sense refers to the three Olympic lifts, which are all overhead lifts.

Power lifting, something I don't really get into here, encompasses such lifts as the bench press and the dead lift. These became popular later—really taking off in the '70s—and are more commonly used in bodybuilders' training than is traditional weight lifting.

The terms *gymnastics* and *acrobatics* are fairly interchangeable as used here in this book. Most of the Muscle Beach athletes who practiced gymnastics were actually practicing the branch of gymnastics known as acrobatics. Both encompass a range of activities. Gymnastic sports such as the parallel bars, high rings, and tumbling (mat work) are Olympic competition sports. Hand balancing, which is part of the acrobatics subset, is not. In general, I use the term *gymnastics* as an umbrella term, to refer to the Olympic sports. *Acrobatics* more often refers to an exhibition staged for entertainment purposes and usually describes group rather than solo routines.

In a broad sense, according to Muscle Beach alumna and acrobatics expert Paula Unger Boelsems, acrobatics encompasses a very broad range of activities, from diving to ice-skating to routines done on a trampoline. In this sense, acrobatics also probably encompasses many of the "extreme" sports popular with young people today, as exemplified in the recently launched X Games.

Adagio is a specific term used by the acrobats of Muscle Beach to define a type of lyrical gymnastic "dance," in which one person (usually a woman) is tossed into the air and caught (usually by a man) in graceful positions.

Finally, bodybuilding today is a professional sport with its own evolving, somewhat subjective, set of aesthetic criteria. It is not an Olympic sport. When I call someone a bodybuilder, it means he worked on developing his body according to the standards of his or her time. The early bodybuilders will quickly admit they'd be dwarfed by today's bodybuilders, who commonly take steroids to add huge amounts of muscle mass.

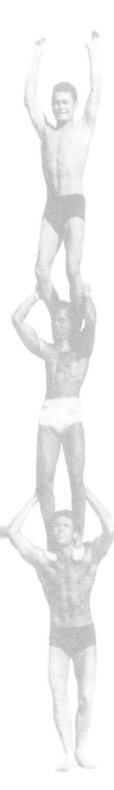

1

Exhibitionists: The Beginnings of Muscle Beach

Muscle Beach is a famous name today world-wide, but it is especially so in Southern California. Santa Monica alone is home to Muscle Beach Burgers, the Muscle Beach Café, and Muscle Beach Hair and Nail Salon. Visit the greater Los Angeles area—from the boardwalk souvenir stands in Venice to the gift shops along down-at-the-heels Hollywood Boulevard—and you'll find postcards, T-shirts, and keychains with the name emblazoned on them.

Many of the items are cheesy, emphasizing sexy cheese- and beefcake over athleticism ("Muscle Beach, California" postcards featuring suggestive photos of thong-clad women or leering, buff men). Few people today seem to know what Muscle Beach really was. In our prepackaged world, it's easier to grasp the simplified idea of a place where buff men went to lift weights and pick up girls. There was some of that, of course, but it was infinitely more rich. In generalizing, we lose the unique individuals on which accurate, three-dimensional history is based.

The reason we think Muscle Beach was a bunch of muscular men lifting weights is because that's what it largely became in later years—after the acrobats who had made up the tapestry of Muscle Beach's first decade moved on. But before that, it was a much different place.

Muscle Beach in its heyday was made up of men, women, and children who were learning, performing, and teaching athletic feats, to the delight of thousands of people. It was a place where rank amateurs could learn from each other and from professionals who were passing through town, and emerge as world-class athletes, stuntmen, Mr. Americas. It was a remarkable, outdoor, public training ground for some of the best all-around athletes America has ever produced. It also became an incubator for some of the country's most influential fitness entrepreneurs: Jack LaLanne and Vic Tanny were just two of the many who made names for themselves there. And yes, there were buff musclemen and the beautiful, buxom, women who loved them.

All this existed on the beach, in the shadow of one of the great amusement piers of its time: the Santa Monica Pier. Families and people of all ages would come to play in the surf, have a hot dog, and watch the folks of Muscle Beach put on a remarkable, day-long show. They could even join in if they wanted, trying a handstand or a balancing act.

The athletes of Muscle Beach literally changed their lives through exercise, and, in turn, changed the world around them. Many of them were children of poor immigrants, who found their version of the American dream through pumping iron. Others were corn-fed Americans, who changed just as dramatically through their pursuits as the immigrants' sons.

If you had come to Muscle Beach on, say, July 4, 1948, you

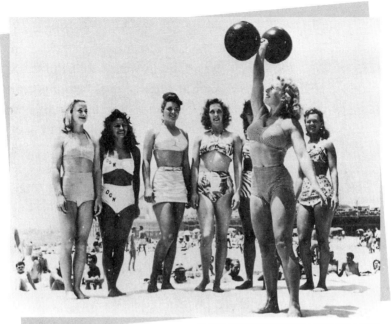

PUDGY STOCKTON LIFTING A DUMBBELL WITH
ONE ARM. LOOKING ON ARE (FROM LEFT)
RELNA BREWER MCRAE, DOLLY WALKER,
JACKIE MCCULLOUGH, LISLE DELAMATER,
MARIAN ZINKIN (HIDDEN), AND VERA FREID.

would have witnessed quite a scene. Several thousand people
would have been jamming the area all around Muscle Beach:
many of the men properly dressed for the times in shirtsleeves,
slacks, and straw hats; women in plaid shirts, cotton pants, and
coordinating head scarves. A number of the spectators may have
been former GIs, who had fallen in love with Southern California when they passed through during the war, and later moved
there with their young families as soon as they could.

The fine, white sand was all but invisible, hidden by a sea of
colorful swim outfits and beach umbrellas. Early arrivals had
claimed seats on the benches that faced the raised Muscle Beach
platform, long before the festivities began. The beach was lined
with snack shops, though many budget-conscious beachgoers
brought their own picnics to spread out on the sand.

By early afternoon, several dozen gymnasts, bodybuilders, and weight lifters would have been entertaining the crowd. Professional stuntmen and circus performers were among those onstage. Acrobats would form human pillars, three and four people high, to amuse the crowd. They would do flips and handstands; a brave and brazen few would even go on the rooftops of buildings overlooking the beach, and perform their handstands there on the edges of roofs while the crowd gasped and hollered.

Several strong women might have come out to lift weights, tear phone books in half, and even "wrestle" with men using martial arts techniques. Girls as young as ten would be part of accomplished teams performing "adagio," a kind of acrobatic dance. Others would support adults several times their own body weight on their backs.

The crowning event was the Mr. and Miss Muscle Beach physique contests, with the winners receiving gleaming trophies that were several feet high. The crowd would whoop and whistle for their favorites. No doubt, a number of Southern California kids developed their first serious crushes on the bronzed Adonises and Venuses who won those awards.

Muscle Beach's reach extended far beyond Los Angeles, though, through pictures and traveling exhibitions put on by people from its community. Its reach ultimately extended around the world, to millions of people. By the '50s, fans and followers worldwide would write to the stars of Muscle Beach, addressing their letters simply to "Muscle Beach, U.S.A." The post office knew where to make the delivery: bags full of mail would arrive at the beach each week.

Little of this history is remembered by present-day Angelenos. Even in Muscle Beach's backyard, the image of Muscle Beach is simplistic and hazy. A "new" Muscle Beach in Santa Monica, opened in the fall of 1999, barely does the original justice. In fact, children are barred from using much of the equipment there, and no weights are allowed. Even sunny weekend afternoons often find the place deserted.

What happened? Decades have passed, and the story of the beach has been clouded by the years and by controversy. Memories among the old-timers with regard to who was there first and when it all started vary widely, as do their versions of the events that led to the closing of Muscle Beach in the late '50s.

There is no escaping today's emphasis on a beefcake image of Muscle Beach. Part of it is guilt by association. It is true that a significant number of enthusiasts for photographs and exhibitions related to fitness has always been those with what might be euphemistically called "impure thoughts." It's also true that the audience for photographs of muscular male nudes was catered to by a handful of periodicals by the early 1950s. Some of these magazines, with such titles as *Physique Pictorial, Vim, Grecian Guild Pictorial,* and *Adonis* (the latter published by fitness entrepreneur Joe Weider), tested—and sometimes overstepped—the strict limits of United States law at the time. Whereas "girlie" magazines at the time pictured soft, rounded women, the men's magazine emphasized Grade A, highly developed beef.

Publishers of these periodicals faced an uphill battle, often running afoul of strict censorship laws. Not only was male frontal nudity verboten, so were the crack between the buttocks and any pictures that were judged to be purely titillating in nature.

Though the core members of Muscle Beach were not involved in the seamier side of the world of nude photography, where many models were hustlers and small-time criminals, some did pose for "artful" nude shots. Unfortunately, as the 1950s went on, many legitimate musclemen suffered from guilt by association by those who scorned the soft-core porn physique magazines of the day.

Most of the Muscle Beach athletes didn't take part in this world. Plenty of flirting and dating that actually led to marriages came out of the socializing between the men and women at Muscle Beach. Certainly, the men liked to impress the pretty girls in the audience. But it was pretty much on the up-and-up, as they would have said in those days.

A number of the people of Muscle Beach, both male and female, admit they received a number of propositions in their day. These ranged from all-expense-paid "visits" to well-heeled fans in faraway places to inducements of hundreds of dollars in exchange for posing for nude photos. Such offers were, as a general rule, turned down flat.

Still, there has always been a connection between images of strong, healthy bodies and sex. This has been the case for millennia—the average person doesn't see sexually explicit paintings and sculptures from ancient times on display in museums, but they exist in back rooms and private collections. In modern times, it's been in evidence from the turn of the century, when photographs of naked men and women in classical poses became popular on "French"-type postcards, to the present day, when you can buy illicit videotapes of athletes in locker rooms. Incidentally, an Internet search today for "Muscle Beach" yields numerous references to pornographic Web sites—virtually all unconnected to the real Muscle Beach.

Certainly, there was a small amount of crossover between the athletes at Muscle Beach and the shadowy world of mostly gay-oriented physique photography. In the book *Beefcake* by F. Valentine Hooven III and the 1999 movie of the same name, it's pointed out that Jack LaLanne, for example, posed for the same photographers who peddled nude male photos by mail in the 1940s. Some of these photographers no doubt visited Muscle Beach, to try to recruit models.

No matter who their audience was, those in the fitness movement itself have often used sex as a selling point in pitches for

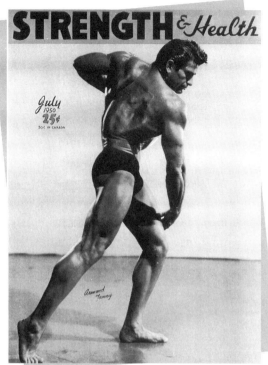

STRENGTH & Health

July
1950
25¢
30¢ IN CANADA

Armand
Tanny

ARMAND TANNY ON THE
COVER OF *STRENGTH &
HEALTH*, 1950.

everything from "energy" potions to gyms. From the earliest days of the "modern" health-spa-type gyms, sex has been a greater motivator than health in getting people in the door.

"When the [Tanny] gyms were in operation, we did a survey," recalled Armand Tanny, a former Mr. America who was brother to and, for a time, the business partner of early gym mogul Vic Tanny. "We found that the main reason for working out was not for health, but for looking good. That," he added with a smile, "was among both men and women, I might add."

So it shouldn't come as a surprise that as far back as the 1930s, stuck among the more lurid magazines on newsstands—alongside the tabloid rags covering movie-star scandals and "true crime" stories—were a number of titles covering "physical culture." That's what they called fitness in those days; it was considered a scientific study of the human body rather than just a quest for physical perfection.

Bernarr Macfadden's *Physical Culture* and Bob Hoffman's *Strength & Health* were the leaders. *Iron Man* was started in 1936 by school custodian Peary Rader and outlived most of the others. But at least forty other physical-culture magazines are estimated to have debuted in the 1930s. Most folded due to low subscription rates and financial woes. As is the case today, publishers in those days found it was hard to make a stand-alone magazine profitable. The most successful found ways to capitalize on related products—often promoting athletic contests that would draw sponsors, and endorsing and selling fitness-related items.

The physical culture magazines' proximity to the more scandalous fare on the newsstand was no accident: Macfadden also published such titles as *True Story,* the first of the "confessional" magazines. In a way, publishers like Macfadden were providing the print equivalent of the tabloid TV shows of our time.

Like fitness gurus before and since, Macfadden was a genius of showmanship and hard-nosed salesmanship. Even those who acknowledge his great influence on the fitness movement often label him a "huckster." His fitness motto was blunt: "Weakness Is a Crime, Don't Be a Criminal."

Their grainy pictures of muscular men—and, particularly in *Physical Culture*'s case, cheesecake-y cover renderings of toned, scantily clad women—were often considered indecent at the time. Moreover, what the magazines espoused—working out with weights—was still very much frowned upon by mainstream society and the medical establishment, for both sexes.

"Doctors told men . . . they'd get 'musclebound'—or wouldn't be able to get an erection. They told women they'd look like men," recalled early fitness guru Jack LaLanne. In 1936,

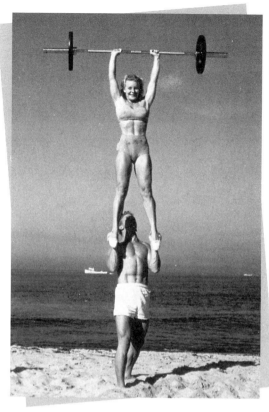

LES STOCKTON HOISTING
A BARBELL-LIFTING PUDGY
STOCKTON ON SANTA
MONICA BEACH, CIRCA
1949.

LaLanne founded his first gym in Oakland, California—across the bay from San Francisco—and became a regular visitor to Muscle Beach. He ended up spreading his fame through television and a nationwide chain of gyms bearing his name, and with the famous media-ready birthday stunts that showcased various feats of strength.

Les and "Pudgy" Stockton, who would become one of Muscle Beach's most famous couples, also recall those days when weight training was practically verboten. When Les attended UCLA, the weights there "were locked in a room that was only accessible to special people . . . too 'dangerous' for general use," said Pudgy.

Modesty was also a consideration: people in polite society did not wear formfitting outfits. Though skirts had gotten much shorter in the '20s, they were still relatively loose fitting. In a way, the "flapper" dresses actually de-emphasized the female form, since a flat chest (sometimes achieved by more buxom girls by taping their breasts down) was part of the look.

There were still many fashions that were considered beyond the pale in the 1930s. For example, in the mid-1930s, only at the beach and only among more liberal types were topless men's suits and skirtless women's suits accepted. Pudgy recalls a young woman she worked with at that time whose husband unequivocally forbade her to wear a swimsuit she'd bought because it didn't have the requisite little skirt in front. "We all got a chuckle out of that," Pudgy admits.

If there was one place in America where the scandalous was practically mundane, it was Los Angeles. The city always had a conservative element, but the best they could do to stave off the inevitable encroachment of showfolk was to try to ban them from their country clubs and social groups. Meanwhile, movie stars like Charlie Chaplin and Fatty Arbuckle continued to make headlines with their bad behavior.

By the 1920s Los Angeles had firmly established itself as a place that attracted offbeat types from the four corners of the earth. Every type of physical, mental, or religious philosophy seemed to be represented in L.A. in greater numbers than just about anywhere else; they catered to the entertainment crowd and to the thousands of others flocking to California to chase their dreams.

The proximity of flesh-worshiping Hollywood, coupled with mild weather that lent itself to year-round outdoor activity, created a perfect breeding ground for the physical-fitness boom. Muscle Beach would become part old-time revival meeting, part infomercial—and all show business.

Actually, the foundations of the fitness movement, including weight lifting and gymnastics, came primarily from Europe. The old country had a much more deep-seated tradition of these kinds of sports. Beginning in the Renaissance, Europeans rediscovered basic tenets of fitness as it was practiced in ancient times.

The rediscovered pursuit of fitness moved ahead by fits and starts from the Renaissance through the early 1900s. Inventors came up with crude dumbbells and even cast-iron crowns meant to strengthen the neck muscles, but they would go by the wayside due to their cost or impracticality. It wasn't until the Industrial Revolution was in full swing, producing useful materials for equipment building and bringing a greater concentration of people to cities where gymnastics and other fitness pursuits would become popularized, that the progress of fitness began to move forward in a fairly straight line.

Nineteenth-century America was only a century removed from being a totally agrarian nation, with few big cities. Weight lifting and gymnastics first started taking hold in the mid-1800s on the East Coast, and remained largely confined there until the second or third decade of the twentieth century.

But it was on the beaches of Southern California, decades later, that the various strains of sports enthusiasm combined to create a truly American fitness movement. Acrobats, stuntmen, weight lifters, and other "health nuts" found common ground at Muscle Beach.

The qualities that led to the success of the American muscle movement included its emphasis on individual achievement and the sheer size and zeal of the athletes themselves. In a land of cowboys, the musclemen became the ultimate cowboys: charming and intensely physical yet aloof and untouchable, idealized, and admired by all.

. . .

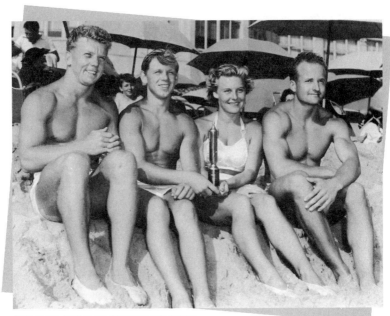

AT THE DEL MAR CLUB: (LEFT TO RIGHT) LES
STOCKTON, GLENN "WHITEY" SUNDBY,
PUDGY STOCKTON, AND JACK MARLOW,
HOLDING A TROPHY FOR THEIR PHYSICAL
FEATS. (A.P. GRIFFITH)

Today, sixty-plus years since the place got its start, the name
Muscle Beach still has a mythic quality that has far outlived its
twenty-five-year existence in Santa Monica, California. Over
the years, there have been other attractions and physique contests up and down the coast—and surely around the world—that
have borrowed the moniker.

Muscle Beach defined the tanned and toned image of Southern California on film and in print, decades before TV shows
such as *Baywatch,* which also use the Santa Monica Beach locale.
That's surely a major reason for the staying power of the Muscle
Beach name: it sums up, in a nutshell, what fitness came to represent in Los Angeles, and what the place in turn reflected back
to the world in a thousand movies, photographs, and postcards.

The name Muscle Beach was an invention of outsiders—not
those who congregated at the area of the Santa Monica Beach

Playground, where Muscle Beach was founded. Between about 1932 and 1934, the core athletes assembled. Eventually, a platform was erected, acrobats arrived, and the place was christened Muscle Beach.

Some young people started working out at the beach informally, using rugs and tarps laid directly on the sand. Within a couple of years, a low wooden platform was built. That was replaced by a sturdier, raised platform, and still later the fully formed, L-shaped platform with its own equipment shed and rows of benches to accommodate spectators.

The beginning—like the end—of Muscle Beach remains a subject of some controversy among old-timers. It is a point of pride to be able to claim to have been among the first to arrive. Muscle Beach alumni disagree about whether it was 1934, 1932, or even earlier when the first young people who became the core of the Muscle Beach crowd started frequenting the area.

What does seem clear is that the area that became known as Muscle Beach had, until at least the mid-1930s, been called High School Beach because of its close proximity to Santa Monica High School, which was built in the 1920s. Some referred to the stretch a mile or so north, favored by University of California at Los Angeles students, as Brain Beach.

Working out on the sand wasn't a completely novel idea. Around the United States and Canada, there were a few beaches that were already the scene of some limited acrobatic activities. The beach provided a free, spacious, easy place to work out. The sand provided built-in padding to break falls. In the absence of a suitable gym, it was often the best place in town to work out.

Down the coast from the pier in Santa Monica, the wrestlers, circus folk, and vaudeville performers who lived in the area or made frequent visits there with their shows were already congregating at Crystal Beach, near the Crystal Pier. Vaudeville was still very active in L.A. through the mid-1930s; there were several first-tier vaudeville theaters in downtown Los Angeles.

There were a couple of big venues for wrestling and boxing not far from the beach. Even then, wrestling was quite a popular diversion, with story lines, good guys, and bad guys—just like today. And there was a circus in town nearly every month. Live entertainment thrived.

Crystal Beach was halfway between the Santa Monica and Ocean Park (South Santa Monica) piers, and was home to a famous bathhouse. "This was way before the Santa Monica Muscle Beach—Crystal Beach," recalled the late Frank Jares, a wrestler who was interviewed by his sportswriter son Joe Jares years later. "Down on the beach on Sundays was a continual workout."

Early Muscle Beach gymnast Ran (short for Randall) Hall also recalled the early activity in that area. "In those days," he wrote in an issue of the *Muscle Beach Alumni Association Newsletter*, "vaudeville was still active in the downtown theaters, especially the five-a-day at the Orpheum, the Million Dollar theater, the Hippodrome, and also the Strand in Long Beach.

"The various acts would visit the gym [at the downtown Los Angeles Athletic Club, which for years was L.A.'s premier gym]," continued Hall, "and work out between shows. They also found a spot at the beach where they could sun and relax and work out too. This was north of the pier at Ocean Park."

Hall names 1932 as the year the future Muscle Beach became a spot for gymnastics. That was the year the Olympic games came to town, a big event that inspired some of the local kids to take up or become more serious about gymnastics. He says that he, Johnny Collins—an East Los Angeles–born acrobat who literally ran away to join the circus as a boy and would become a founding member of the Muscle Beach crowd—and several others were alternating between the Ocean Park/Crystal Beach area and the Santa Monica pier area by that time in 1932.

Certainly, the performers and wrestlers who had already been congregating on the beach a little further south attracted some spectators. Hall admits he was "starstruck," and used to go to Ocean Park "just to mingle" with the pros. But this scene never became as big as Muscle Beach would become.

They didn't really set out to stage one of the greatest ongoing gymnastics shows the world has ever seen. But the place took hold and took off with spectators within a few short years. By the early 1940s, with the area then widely known for its gymnastics exhibitions and well-built inhabitants, visitors to the beach in the sleepy, conservative town had dubbed the place Muscle Beach. Some say the name even had a slightly derisive connotation—muscle equating with all brawn, no brain. But it was catchy, and it stuck. Another theory, that the place was originally known as Muscle Beach, and that *muscle* was a play on words, seems unlikely.

Regardless of the name's origin, visitors who came upon Muscle Beach loved it. It was a constant show, an adjunct to the nearby amusement destinations of the Santa Monica and Crystal Piers. It was yet another form of spontaneous, live entertainment. Unlike many of the ocean-front entertainments, it was absolutely free.

Muscle Beach didn't reach the full height of its international fame until the postwar boom years, when everything seemed to become outsized. But it got a nudge in the quieter days of the Depression—thanks in part, in true California fashion, to a teenager and an earthquake.

Paul Brewer was a sixteen-year-old student at Santa Monica High School in 1934. He learned some gymnastics skills in junior high: tumbling, ring work, and the like. Like many young people, he was probably inspired in part by the 1932 summer Olympic games in Los Angeles, where gymnastics were showcased.

But when he got to Santa Monica High, Brewer's athletic ambitions were frustrated. The school's plans for a boys' gymnasium were put on hold following the Long Beach earthquake in March 1933. There wasn't an adequate facility for him and his fellow classmates to work out in.

The quake was a big setback to the entire city, not just to one boy's dreams. All told, nearly 120 people were killed and $50 million in losses were attributed to the quake. Due to structural damage, "Samo High" became a "tent city" for months.

The only equipment Brewer and his classmates had to work out on was a horizontal bar, parallel bars, and a horizontal ladder (the raised apparatus one crosses by swinging from hand to hand) in a sandpit outside the boys' locker room. It wasn't enough to satisfy the young gymnast.

On the weekends and after classes in 1934, Brewer, friend Jimmy Pfeiffer, and several other classmates gravitated toward the biggest sandpit in town: Santa Monica Beach, just four blocks from the school. In addition to a handful of other young acrobats apparently establishing a beachhead there, some very basic playground equipment was already in place.

A few years earlier, it seems, a Santa Monica recreational worker and mother named Kate Giroux had gotten the city, along with some help from the Depression-era Works Project Administration, to install some children's playground equipment near the popular Santa Monica Pier. According to Ran Hall, there was already some activity there starting in 1932. Other accounts closer to the actual time say that young athletes would occasionally use the playground for a workout as far back as the mid-1920s.

The very first children's equipment there was installed in 1925. The collection of equipment—including such basics as swings and a slide—was called the Santa Monica Beach Playground. There were kiddie-themed horizontal ladders, sized for "mama bear," "papa bear," and "baby bear." Not exactly the training equipment of champions.

Some of the young gymnasts had earlier tried to get the city of Santa Monica to install more adult equipment in the area—and had been rebuffed. There was some prejudice against people who were considered "show-offs" or "exhibitionists" at the beach. A 1938 article in the *Los Angeles Times Sunday Magazine* explained:

> The Beach is usually thought to be a place where game playing and acrobatics are a public nuisance. The average citizen is all too familiar with that unnecessary variety of the genus beachgoer who insists upon doing a shaky handstand within easy falling distance of his neighbors or who struts and bulges his muscles for the amazement of his more *normal* [my italics] brethren.

In the wake of the earthquake and with the Depression at its depths, though, the city relented. Kids needed something to do, and this proposal seemed relatively harmless. City officials approved the installation of more equipment, providing the project didn't cost much and was properly supervised. That's where Al Neiderman came in: he was a gymnastics buff in his twenties who worked as a mechanic for the Santa Monica City Bus Company. He would help the Santa Monica students turn the area into a makeshift gym.

At first, they were only allowed to put down a rug for tumbling, right on the sand—very basic stuff. No platform, no fancy equipment, no weights. Just the carpeting, barely long and wide enough to perform some stunts on.

Despite some resistance from recreation workers who wanted to keep the playground strictly for little kids, the group got the go-ahead to add more iron playground equipment, such as parallel bars and high rings. Neiderman lent his tools and welding skills to the operation. Brewer recalled vividly, years later, that he was so anxious to try out the newly erected parallel bars that he burned his leg on a still-hot weld in his rush to be the first one on.

Soon, the students were joined by others, including UCLA gymnastics coach Cece Hollingsworth and his students. Hall remembers Bert Goodrich as a frequent visitor to the beach when he was in town. Goodrich, an Arizona native who would go on to become the first Mr. America in 1939, had been a track and gymnastics star in high school.

After graduation, Goodrich became a performer. First, he was part of a two-man act that toured with circuses and the vaudeville circuit. The story goes that his body was so well developed from his track, gymnastics, and acrobatic training that he really didn't train per se for the Mr. America contest: he just walked in, showed off his body, and won. Later, he became a stand-in for such athletes-turned-movie-stars as Buster Crabbe (the swimmer who was tapped to play Tarzan) and Red Grange (an ex-football hero who got into movies).

Hollingsworth, understanding the importance of community relations between the young gymnasts and Santa Monica, encouraged goodwill between the athletes and the city from the beginning. True to its small-town atmosphere, Santa Monica hosted an annual parade to celebrate "Pioneer Days." Hollingsworth organized his charges at Muscle Beach to build a float that he designed, containing a small tumbling area and a horizontal bar.

For several years starting in the mid-1930s, the float became a popular addition to the parade. The float made its way down Santa Monica streets with young athletes on board, dressed up as pioneer settlers and Indians, performing acrobatic feats—sometimes barely missing trees and power lines as they leapt and flew through the air.

Meanwhile, with the addition of acrobatics, the beach playground became a lot more popular. According to the 1938 *Los Angeles Times Sunday Magazine* article referred to earlier, attendance at the playground jumped more than 500-fold—from 3,500 visitors to 1.8 million—from its opening year to 1938, the fourth year the gymnasts had come down in force.

A 1938-vintage photograph printed with the article shows scores of men, women, and children—sitting, squatting, and standing—gathered around the slim mat running lengthwise toward the ocean that then served as the staging area for Muscle Beach. Later platforms would run parallel to the ocean to accommodate more spectators. The article, notably, did not refer to the place as Muscle Beach yet. That became more common in 1939 and 1940.

Though Santa Monica was a small quiet city, it was a favorite of tourists and Los Angeles residents seeking weekend relaxation. Santa Monica Beach was a long stretch of broad white beach that was easily accessible by car and by the fast, inexpensive electric trolley system that traversed most of L.A. at the time. Its shoreline and endless array of amusements provided a welcome respite to hard-working Angelenos, in the days before home air-conditioning and television.

At that time, few people could afford to take a real vacation to distant beaches. It was considered a real treat for people from all around the area to come to Santa Monica for the day, put up an umbrella on the sand, and eat a picnic lunch. The seashore was mobbed with people doing just that on summer weekends.

The pier was one of several along a two-mile stretch of beach from Santa Monica to Venice. Venice's pier, the southernmost, had more of a down-market, "carny" atmosphere. Venice—which had been planned as a city modeled after the Italian city, complete with canals and gondolas—had seen its heyday in the early 1920s, but had since steadily declined as a tourist destina-

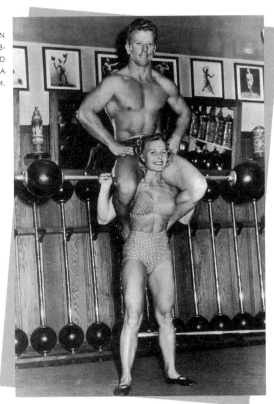

tion. The Venice theme was largely abandoned; canals were filled in or never completed, though a few still exist to this day.

A little further north was the Ocean Park Pier, which became a popular amusement-park attraction, featuring arcades and rides. Just to the north of it was the slightly fancier Crystal Pier, home to the popular Crystal Ballroom and a number of eateries.

Santa Monica's was the most upscale and family-friendly of the piers. According to Fred Basten in *Santa Monica Bay: Paradise by the Sea*: "With Ocean Park and Venice taking up the 'carnival spirit,' Santa Monica began emphasizing ease of living, the quiet home life and pleasant and cultural surroundings." In other words, it wasn't the most likely place for a big, brash, crowd-drawing attraction like Muscle Beach to take hold.

Muscle Beach was founded by beginners, but they would quickly learn and attract more accomplished athletes to join in the action there. There was no shortage of world-class acrobats coming through Los Angeles at any given time in the 1930s.

At that time, nightclub acts featuring acrobatics—a close cousin to the gymnastics practiced by the UCLA students—were very popular. Acrobatics encompassed separate disciplines, such as hand balancing and tumbling. It was big, showy, and entertaining; audiences could also enjoy acrobats in the numerous vaudeville acts and traveling circuses that passed through L.A. Top acrobatic acts could be headliners, or often opened for top-billed musicians, comedians, and the like. Word spread among professional acts that Muscle Beach was a prime area to practice stunts—just as professional wrestlers had already started to congregate to work out, spar, and socialize at Crystal Beach. It became de rigueur for acts passing through town to make a pilgrimage to the beach.

It was quite a scene. An American flag flew proudly over the equipment shed as the athletes worked out on the platform. Some more daring Muscle Beachers would even take their acts up onto the buildings overlooking the beach and balance on the edge of their rooftops. Even for experienced acrobats, it was a hot-dog, risky move. The audience would gasp as they performed handstands four stories high without a net; even their colleagues would whoop and holler. They loved the attention.

By this time, the "amateurs" who had founded Muscle Beach could barely be distinguished from the professionals. In fact, a number of Muscle Beach graduates went on to form their own well-known touring acts. Professionals performed at the beach free of charge, to the delight of those who just wandered over or who couldn't normally afford to pay to see such entertainment.

Over the years, hundreds of people got the experience of joining the action, if just for a few minutes. Under the watchful supervision of beach regulars, they could learn to do a handstand, or balance on someone's shoulders. Young athletes just learning the ropes would spend literally all day there working out, stopping only for a quick sandwich and a cup of water or milk.

They might buy something to eat from one of the Nature Boys, who brought fresh fruits and nuts to the beach, or from "Crazy Al," the owner of a food stand adjacent to the platform. Al, himself an immigrant from the Middle East, was known for mumbling and cursing about all sorts of racial groups, and for his rather flattering imitation of Hitler. The Muscle Beach denizens, who represented Los Angeles's melting pot of multigenerational Americans, Slavs, Italians, Russians, Jews—you name it—didn't take Al too seriously. The place had its notorious characters, ones you just shrugged off and counted among the rich pageantry of life at Muscle Beach.

Some of those young Muscle Beach folk, who were then forming their own two- and three-person acts, would go on to become influential in various areas of fitness. Jack LaLanne was part of a two-man act with Jim Drinkward. Glenn Sundby, nicknamed "Whitey" by Les Stockton for his very light blond hair, and his sister Dolores were part of a trio that opened for such famous acts as Spike Jones; Sundby would go on to found *International Gymnast* magazine in 1955.

In the mid-1940s, Les and Abbye "Pudgy" (for her stocky build as a child) Stockton would travel with Mr. Americas Steve Reeves and George Eiferman from New York to Hawaii, putting

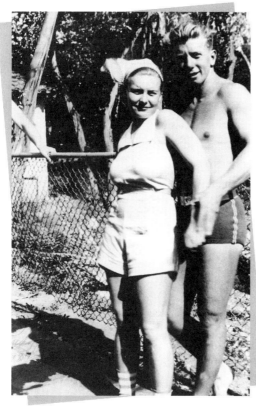

on exhibitions. The Stocktons would go on to found gyms and Pudgy would write on fitness for national magazines; Eiferman would become a frequent lecturer on fitness to school groups; Reeves would become Hercules on the big screen, capitalizing on his phenomenal build and handsome face. In fact, those who knew him in his pre-screen-star days say he was so good-looking that everyone already figured he was a movie star anyway.

LaLanne would launch the first major television fitness show, which aired for more than thirty years. He went on the air locally out of San Francisco in 1951, and nationally from Hollywood in 1959.

These activities all encouraged the spread of the fitness movement as we know it today. It all started with some kids looking for a place to work out on the sand. That place, next to a children's playground, grew from a rug to a rug over a low wooden platform to a raised platform to a raised platform featuring dozens of top-notch performers. Soon, spectators would fill and overflow the rows of benches that were added alongside the platform, like parishioners sitting in pews in a temple to the human form. They were witnessing history in the guise of popular entertainment. Within a few years, it grew into a phenomenon that showcased and encouraged an enormous surge in interest in fitness in America.

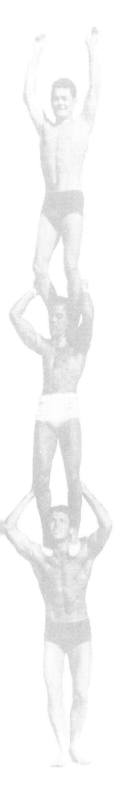

2

The Muscle Comes to Muscle Beach

When did Muscle Beach get its legendary name? Paul Brewer and his sister Relna, who would also become a star at Muscle Beach, believe it happened around the time that Armand and Vic Tanny came to the beach—in 1939 to 1940. These two handsome and famous muscle-men soon attracted other weight-lifting and body-building enthusiasts with them—and the crowds followed.

These guys were big: not just muscular, but massive by the standards of the day. Next to the slender gymnasts, they appeared even bigger. They were like the sideshow strongmen of yes-teryear, gods come down from Mount Olympus to walk among mere mortals. Unlike the old-time strongmen, though, men like the Tannys didn't even need to heft heavy barbells to impress crowds: the very sight of their toned, tanned, and rippling muscles was a show on its own. They were an important element in Muscle Beach's rise in popularity and fame.

Vic Tanny, older by about eight years, would go on to become the more famous of the brothers through his national chain of gyms. But Armand was actually the more accomplished athlete. He arrived in Santa Monica first, from the Tannys' hometown of Rochester, New York.

Growing up on the East Coast, the two Italian-American boys had become interested in weight lifting. They avidly read magazines like Bob Hoffman's influential *Strength & Health*. Vic got into it first; he encouraged Armand to start lifting weights at the age of twelve. By the time he was eighteen, Armand Tanny was "pretty much national caliber," he recalls matter-of-factly.

The Tannys became known for their strong builds, but for years "nobody in school really knew what I was up to," Armand says. That changed in his senior year, when young Armand—hoping to spread the word on weight training, and probably to gain some adulation in the process—offered to put on a weight-lifting exhibition at a school assembly.

The show was a hit. His classmates, who may have seen strongmen hoist weights at the circus but had no idea there was one among them, were bowled over. "After that, I was a school hero," Tanny says with a laugh.

Armand was also a good student. He'd become interested in science and medicine partly through his athletic pursuits, and decided to major in premedical studies in college. He enrolled at the University of Rochester, in his hometown. He figured he'd save a little money by living at home, and study hard to become a doctor. That was the all-American dream, especially for a young man in a family of recent immigrants.

Vic, meanwhile, had become a schoolteacher. One summer in the late 1930s he visited Southern California with a couple of buddies. He'd been hearing a lot about California; beginning in the 1920s, the state had started aggressively promoting the Southland as an ideal place to settle. Plenty of cheap land and year-round sunshine, the ads boasted. In the Golden State, Tanny too found paradise: more sun, sand, and pretty girls in one place than he'd ever known existed.

Vic convinced Armand that the West Coast was the place to be. Not only could he go to the state-run UCLA for a fraction of the cost of the University of Rochester, he would be in sunny California and in the heart of its burgeoning fitness scene. He told Armand to go ahead to California while he finished up his teaching year. "I'll come out to join you next year," Vic promised.

Armand was accepted into UCLA, which cost about ten percent of what Rochester did for a term—$35, versus $300. That alone made it an obvious choice for the young student. Armand got on a cross-country bus. At the end of his long ride, he settled near UCLA's Westwood campus, a short drive from the beach.

Armand didn't really know about the Muscle Beach scene, though. He figured that moving to Los Angeles was a trade-off: He "didn't think they knew much about weight lifting out here anyway," he recalled. He figured he'd be busy with his studies, anyway. He thought only people on the East Coast were into weights.

But the week after Tanny's bus rolled into town, he and thousands of other Angelenos were hitting the beaches. The city was in the grip of a near-record heat wave; temperatures stayed up around 100 degrees, even at night. Tanny was lounging on the beach north of Santa Monica Pier, when he heard a familiar clattering noise.

"I thought, gee, that sounds like a barbell," he said, remembering. He walked in the direction of the sound, toward the pier, and soon came upon the Santa Monica Beach Playground.

There, because the heat was drawing people onto the beach later into the evening than usual, a dozen or more Muscle Beach regulars were going about their usual routine. They were lifting weights, swinging on the high bars, doing fly-away leaps off the rings.

Tanny's strong, square jaw nearly dropped to the ground. "I was totally impressed," Tanny recalled, still amazed at the memory of discovering the place. "I sat there late into the night. I went back the next day and the next day, and got involved in all the activities there."

Armand brought his weight-lifting and wrestling buddies from UCLA as well. Some of these men weren't just working out with weights to strengthen their bodies for gymnastics. They were actively building their bodies, striving to achieve more muscle mass and size than the next guy. They were among the earliest bodybuilders, a new breed. Not strongmen, not weight lifters, but people whose goal was to create the ideal body.

That year, 1939, marked the very first Mr. America contest, under the auspices of the Amateur Athletic Union (later, financial backers would create a "professional" Mr. America competition; these early titles are referred to as "amateur" Mr. Americas). Bodybuilding as a distinct sport was really born that year. The contest was won by none other than Bert Goodrich, the ex-circus performer and Muscle Beach regular. Goodrich would become Tanny's brother-in-law within a few years when he married Armand's sister.

In addition to being noticeably bigger than most of the other men at the beach, Armand Tanny was tanned and handsome, with a shock of shiny black hair and what people would come to call a "million-dollar smile." Along with his friends, including brother Vic who arrived in 1940, he helped earn the place the name Muscle Beach.

Armand Tanny was a smart, accomplished athlete who was skilled at weight lifting, bodybuilding, and wrestling. As the years went on, though, the beach continued to attract newcomers. Many were more concerned with pure physical appearance than they were with learning and performing acrobatic feats, which provoked some resentment on the part of the gymnasts who had put Muscle Beach on the map.

"Over the years I have always tried to contribute to the stature of Muscle Beach," said Ran Hall years later. "I was disappointed when the body builders and no-talent glamour boys and girls started to take over. Until then it was a fraternal group where we taught, learned, experimented, and encouraged each other to develop our talents."

The gymnasts even chafed a bit at the name Muscle Beach. They tended to refer to it as the playground or simply the beach. But it was a losing battle; everyone else latched onto the name Muscle Beach.

Most of the regulars learned to embrace it. "We thought the Muscle Beach identification for the playground was a little sarcastic," remembered Paul Brewer. "But in time," he admitted, "we learned to accept the name as it became world famous."

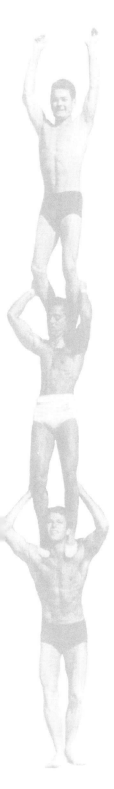

3

The Women of Muscle Beach

When women's bodybuilding became widely popular in the 1980s, many thought that these were pioneers in a man's world—a product of the women's equality movement. More recently, we've been hearing about women wrestling men "for the first time ever," in promotional stunts for professional wrestling.

None of these "firsts" are truly unprecedented. As far back as the 1930s, there were women becoming well known for building up their bodies through weight training, and women who would "wrestle" men in at least as authentic a way as today's female wrestlers do. Muscle Beach, naturally, became a showcase for ideal physiques, both male and female.

In Muscle Beach's first decade—through the 1940s—the area was known for acrobatics rather than the "iron" sports of weight lifting and body-

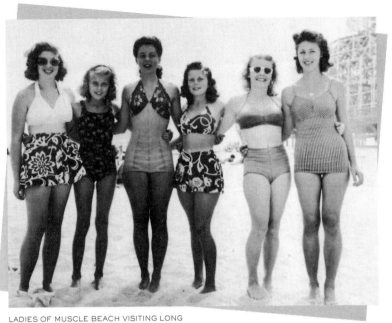

LADIES OF MUSCLE BEACH VISITING LONG
BEACH: *(LEFT TO RIGHT)* TWO UNIDENTIFIED WOMEN,
BETTY CONNER (WIFE OF BRUCE CONNER), AN UNIDEN-
TIFIED FRIEND, PUDGY, AND MARIAN ZINKIN (WIFE OF
HAROLD ZINKIN).

building. The early habitués of Muscle Beach were working out
with weights, but it took a backseat to acrobatic and gymnastic
shows.

Unlike weight lifting, acrobatics relied as much on grace and
skill as on sheer power. Women and even children were active
participants: at Muscle Beach, Paula Unger Boelsems, Relna
Brewer, and Abbye "Pudgy" Stockton became just a few of the
well-known female stars.

Women were considered equals by their male counterparts—
at least on the platform. In acrobatic formations and acts made
up of two or more people, women were well represented at Muscle Beach. Their exhibitions would often even play on stereotypes
of female weakness, to the delight and amazement of spectators.

Stockton and Brewer, younger sister of Muscle Beach cofounder Paul Brewer, would tear books in half onstage and hoist hefty barbells with one hand. Pudgy would lift a man with one hand, or support him on her shoulders. Relna would "wrestle" with men—actually, she would use martial-arts moves to toss them around like rag dolls. Relna wasn't crazy about being called a wrestler, but audiences ate it up. So when there were crowds and photographers around, those folks at the beach who had a nose for publicity made sure she performed her wrestling act.

Even little girls became stars for their feats of strength. Beverly Jocher started coming to the beach at age five, soon after her family moved to Santa Monica from Philadelphia. Trained by Muscle Beach's finest, she was lifting adults by age eight. By age ten, she could balance nearly 400 pounds of adults on her tiny frame. By seventeen, she was supporting 590 pounds of them on her 110-pound body, and became a state weight-lifting champ.

Similarly, preteen April Atkins was hoisting two and three people at a time, whose combined weight exceeded 400 pounds. And Edna Rivers was regarded as the strongest girl ever at the beach. Rivers was a judo whiz and could reportedly lift five women and a man up on a beach board with ease.

These girls grew up around the beach and trained from a very early age. They put to rest the popular belief—which has taken decades to shake—that girls aren't cut out for sports. Quite simply, they were encouraged and taught—rather than being told they were "just girls." And contrary to stereotyping, they grew into beautiful young ladies, not husky Amazons. In addition to her athletic accolades, Jocher would go on to win beauty contests, including Miss Southern California and Miss Pacific Coast.

The ladies became a particular favorite of photographers, who immediately saw the novelty and marketability of chicks with pecs. Newsreel footage of Relna throwing the men around showed up in the Movietone News that ran before films in theaters. Pudgy was the star of such newsreels as "Whatta Build,"

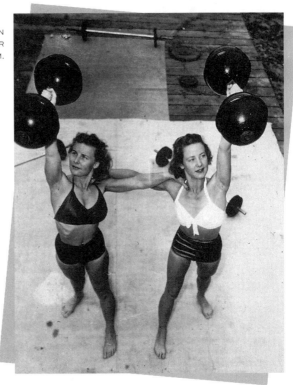

which featured her lifting husband Les over her head with one hand. Lensmen for various newsweeklies, papers, and tabloids, including *Life, Look,* and *Pic,* liked to snap the women flexing their muscles.

Pudgy stopped doing overt, bicep-flexing "muscle" poses for cameramen when she realized such pictures were being used to suggest women became masculine through bodybuilding. In her photos, she would try to emphasize graceful, "feminine" poses, which highlighted her muscularity without making her look like she was trying to compete with the guys when it came to the size of her arm muscles.

On the flip side, bodybuilder and weight lifter Armand Tanny claims he turned down bit parts in movies that would have had him getting beaten up by the skinnier hero. It was typical show biz to want to show muscular women as threatening and muscular men as weak. "I said, 'No way, I don't need that,'" recalls Tanny. Though Tanny did end up doing some work on stage and screen, his biggest contribution to helping dispel myths about weight training would come from his long-running column for *Muscle and Fitness.*

When a local newspaper did a feature on musclewomen Pudgy and Relna in the '40s, the writer and photographer went out of their way to show that the women were "dynamic" but still "dainty" and ladylike. A layout in the *Los Angeles Examiner's* (a now-defunct daily paper) magazine section, the *American Weekly,* pictured the two women lifting dumbbells and performing stunts—alongside photos of Pudgy at home, sewing and washing dishes, smiling in a modest dress and apron. Readers were assured that the status quo remained intact.

The duo became two of the most famous ladies of Muscle Beach and grew as close as sisters. Both had grown up in the area and shared a love of sport and the outdoors. They were both introduced to fitness through their male relatives or boyfriends, but they took to it like naturals and gained their success on their own.

Relna was brought to Muscle Beach when she was about ten by her brother Paul, the area's teenage cofounder. Paul and their mother, a nurse, encouraged Relna to exercise to overcome the injuries she had sustained in a fire when she was a small child. She was frail for several years due to severe burns on her back; stiff scar tissue had formed, making her slightly hunched over. She lost flexibility and some range of motion.

It was a common story: just as early fitness champion Teddy Roosevelt had exercised his way from a frail childhood to robust health in the nineteenth century, many of those who would become famous at Muscle Beach started life as small, weak chil-

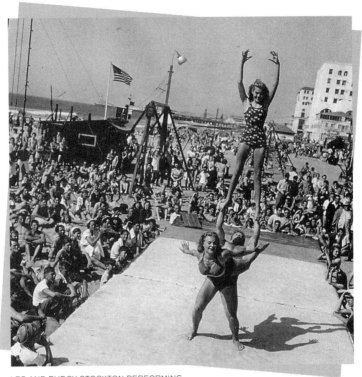

LES AND PUDGY STOCKTON PERFORMING
A STUNT WITH AN UNIDENTIFIED YOUNG LADY.

dren with physical ailments. George Eiferman was born a pree-
mie, and was a small child until he took up weight training.
Glenn Sundby, like Roosevelt, suffered from asthma as a child,
and was frail until he got into gymnastics. The fact that their results were so dramatic only made them more fervent in their
support of exercise. They saw firsthand that exercise and fitness
could make a huge difference in one's health, outlook, and life
in general.

Relna, then, got into exercise with her mother's blessing. Her
mother still made sure she was properly chaperoned at the gym
and the beach, of course, "to protect my reputation," Relna recalled years later with some amusement. She started tagging
along to Muscle Beach with her brother, using the equipment

there to help stretch and strengthen the muscles of her back. She had to start out by just hanging on the bars and letting the scar tissue stretch. After she got to the point where it didn't hurt just to move around normally, Relna started taking classes in physical culture with five other girls at the Elks Club gymnasium in the Ocean Park area of Santa Monica.

Her teacher was Barney Fry, a Douglas Aircraft machinist and an extraordinary amateur athlete. Well into his forties by then, Fry had a knack for developing athletic talent in young people. Boys, girls, it didn't matter to him—he was a firm believer in the benefit of exercise for everyone.

He taught the girls all about diet and exercise. They played basketball and volleyball. They lifted weights and practiced gymnastics. In short, they got a better physical education than most kids (let alone girls) get today.

It was Relna who encouraged Fry to come to Muscle Beach; he would become a fixture there, and a trainer of champions, through the 1950s. He would later teach talented youngsters such as April Atkins and Beverly Jocher the ropes.

As an added bonus, Relna met her future husband, Gordon McRae (no relation to the musical theater star), at the Elks Club gym. She invited him to the beach as well, where he became a frequent visitor and befriended wrestlers like Frank Jares and bodybuilders like Vic Tanny.

Once she started working out with the help of her brother, Fry, and the others at Muscle Beach, Relna discovered she was a born all-around athlete just waiting to blossom. Like a number of Muscle Beachers, she ended up doing a fair amount of movie stunt work—riding horses and falling off cliffs in cowboy movies were among her specialties. Slender, blond, and just five foot two, she could benchpress 150 and dead lift 210. Pretty respectable, and not just "for a girl."

Relna performed feats of strength and trapeze acts with various circus troupes passing through Los Angeles, swam at a World's Fair exhibition, and put in a brief stint as a professional ice skater. Diving, skating, trick riding—they were all forms of the acrobatics Relna had been taught at the beach.

Her wild life settled down rather quickly when she married McRae, who had been a football star in school. "He was afraid I'd break my neck," she explained years later of her retirement from daredevil feats.

Actually, the people of Muscle Beach were extremely proud of their safety record: almost no one taking part in the activities there was seriously hurt over the years. They remember maybe the occasional broken bone, but that was it. Certainly nothing life-threatening. Looking back, many admit with a laugh that it was largely luck—combined, of course, with their skill as practiced athletes.

Of all Muscle Beach's women, Abbye "Pudgy" Stockton became the best known for her remarkable physique, pictured in hundreds of newspapers and magazines during the 1940s. As her friend and fellow weight lifter George Eiferman put it simply, "Pudgy was stacked . . . she was built." She was 38-20-36, to be exact.

Even shorter than Relna at five foot one, Pudgy was muscular and had an ample bosom—a combination difficult for many women to achieve, since breasts are made up of fatty tissue, which is often lost when one starts to train. Naturally, Pudgy attracted many male admirers . . . stares, whistles, besotted fans. Les Stockton good-naturedly admits that he was often jokingly referred to as "Mr. Pudgy."

Abbye was born Abby Eville in Santa Monica; she grew up going to the beach with her outdoors-loving parents. As a child, she earned the nickname "Pudgy" for her solid build. Even af-

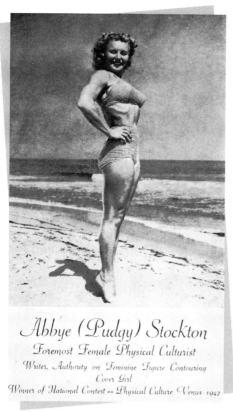

Abbye (Pudgy) Stockton
Foremost Female Physical Culturist
Writer, Authority on Feminine Figure Contouring
Cover Girl
Winner of National Contest ·· Physical Culture Venus 1947

ter her physique became chiseled at Muscle Beach, the name
stuck. She would add the "e" to her first name after marrying
Les; she took the "e" from her maiden name. She figured Abbye
was a little more classy and exotic than Abby.

Besides, people at Muscle Beach changed names the way
other people change their socks. These were show people, many
of them born with somewhat clunky ethnic names, and they
thought nothing of shortening, changing, or enhancing the
names they were given at birth. If their names hadn't already
been chopped off when their families came to the U.S.—like
the Golds and Tannys of the world—they often Americanized
them themselves.

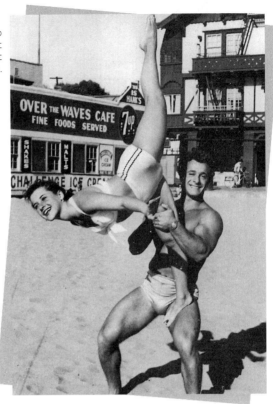

After high school, Pudgy went to work as an operator for the telephone company. Like so many women, she started putting on pounds at her desk job. A photo taken of her shortly before she started working out in the late 1930s shows that, after two years of sitting all day, she was living up to her nickname: she was pretty, but doughy and lacking muscle tone. "I wasn't doing anything at that time but putting on weight," Pudgy says today with a laugh, looking at the photograph.

She also lacked the sparkle and confidence that would soon come with her newly sculpted physique. In the picture taken before she built up her body, she looks shy and hesitant to be photographed. Her head is tilted down, and her hair is pulled straight under a scarf—a far cry from the glamour poses she'd be striking within a couple of years.

Pudgy was encouraged to try weight training by her boyfriend, Les Stockton. He'd taken up weight training himself in his first year at UCLA, along with friend and future gym owner/Muscle Beach colleague Bruce Conner, to add bulk to his slight frame. Pudgy was interested in "reducing," in the lingo of the day, so resisted weight training at first.

She went to the library for tips on exercise, but found virtually nothing. "What there was was pretty hilariously out-of-date" she said, recalling the couple of decades-old manuals on calisthenics she found on the shelves.

One day, Les brought over some light dumbbells. "Just try some exercises," he said. He assured Pudgy that weight training was good for toning and slimming, not just bulking up.

"I was skeptical," admits Pudgy. Most people in those days considered it nearly unthinkable for a woman to work out with weights. But she quickly started to see results and became a convert to physical fitness; she and Les soon became weekend regulars at Muscle Beach.

Pudgy found there were already a number of accomplished women there. Striking, raven-haired sisters Betsy and Kitty Knight had a two-girl acrobatic act, in which they would lift and toss each other into various poses. The Knights were already seasoned professionals, having toured as far afield as Asia with the Marco Show, which featured a very young Danny Kaye as its master of ceremonies and comedian.

Rosie Unger was also frequenting the beach by that time. A skilled gymnast, she was known for her prowess at tumbling from the various gym apparatuses. Rosie's younger sister Paula, like any little sis, was both fascinated by and somewhat jealous of her sister. She pestered her mother to let her go to Muscle Beach, too.

By the age of nine or ten, Paula had started to become a star in her own right, a tiny girl (all of seventy-five pounds, well into her teens) with no fear of being tossed high into the air and caught by other gymnasts. She would become the regular partner of stuntman/acrobat Russ Saunders for years.

The men were a combination of amateur enthusiasts like Les and men who were serious performers/competitors looking for an outlet—movie stuntmen like Saunders and professional acrobats. They welcomed the girls, and were happy to perform with them, teach them, and learn from them.

Men wore basic swim trunks, close-fitting briefs that rose higher on the abdomen than today's Speedo-style trunks. For women, suitable apparel could be a problem. One-piece suits were restrictive. There was no Lycra, no Spandex—let alone two-piece bathing suits for well-endowed women—in those days. Seeing a couple of the other women wearing early versions of bikinis, Pudgy decided to brave it. Her full figure (and, in the beginning, her budget) necessitated a homemade suit.

"My mother ripped apart an old brassiere of mine, and made a pattern from that," recalls Pudgy. The result: a two-piece (modest by our standards today) with a full-coverage top and a brief that rose up to the belly button. In the late 1930s, it was practically grounds for getting arrested. Even into the mid-1950s, it was news in the lifestyle pages when "skintight" swimsuits became fashionable.

On the beach, there was plenty of rubbernecking among the men when Pudgy revealed her busty, curvaceous figure. "Oh sure, the guys did double takes," her husband Les admitted, though he claimed that he took it in stride.

Probably due to the combination of feminine pulchritude and the skill of the athletes, the number of weekend spectators at Muscle Beach was quickly increasing. Benches were added for onlookers next to the platform. Often, audience members of all

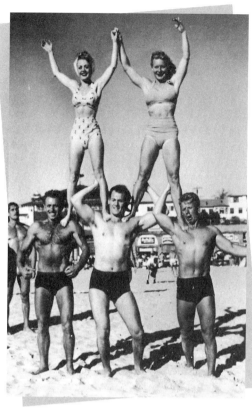

ages would join in, and learn to do a handstand or lift. There could be people of all ages, and both sexes.

The atmosphere certainly had a sexual charge—these were young, extremely attractive (and nearly naked) people. Many regulars ended up meeting their mates working out at the beach and marrying them . . . several repeated this pattern several times, in fact. But it was mainly good, clean fun, with a slight hint of the risqué. "It was the only place you could go in those days and have your hand on the inside of some gal's thigh within five minutes," jokes Les, always ready with a snappy comment.

There wasn't just a fitness revolution in the making. Women were taking a larger public role in society as World War II loomed, then passed. Already, many were entering the workplace; a flood of women would take over traditionally male jobs when the men went off to war.

More and more families, especially in Southern California, were getting automobiles. With cars came mobility, and, of course, greater opportunities for trysts. A 1938 study, quoted in Stephanie Coontz's *The Way We Never Were*, found that two-thirds of women born after 1910 had lost their virginity before marriage—that was up from 26 percent of women who were born between 1890 and 1900. Clearly, a sexual revolution was brewing. Not everyone was comfortable with it. The beautiful, sexy women of Muscle Beach contributed greatly to the beach's rise to international fame. Just as surely, the sexual undertones of the activities there ended up riling some of the more conservative—and powerful—interests in Santa Monica as the years went on.

But the fact that they were there at all, and were successful— early evangelists for women training with weights and building their bodies—is what is remarkable. The story of Muscle Beach's women is one of the most fascinating and overlooked of the many facets of Muscle Beach that have been nearly forgotten by young fitness enthusiasts today.

Fitness historian and writer Jan Todd said in a 1992 article on Pudgy Stockton, "Every woman bodybuilder who puts on a swimsuit and steps up on the posing dais, every woman weight lifter who strains under a clean and jerk, and every woman power lifter who fights through the pull of a heavy dead lift owes a debt of gratitude to Abbye 'Pudgy' Stockton." But even for the majority of women today, who will never perform a lift or pose in a bodybuilding competition, Pudgy and her Muscle Beach sisters were important pioneers. Any woman, in fact, who expects an equal chance in sports, any woman who wants to build her confidence as well as her body through training,

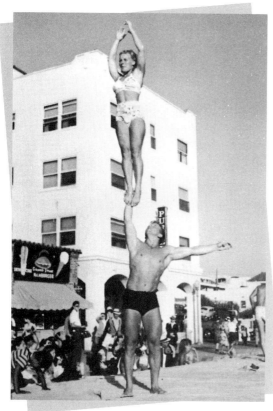

and every woman who thinks female beauty doesn't need to mean being thin and gaunt to be attractive owes them thanks.

For what they demonstrated was not just that women could be strong, powerful, and physically competitive: they, as well as the men of Muscle Beach, showed that the knowledge of and practice of bodybuilding exercise can change lives. It could take a small, scarred little girl and make her a vibrant young woman who wrestled men and performed tricky stunts in movies. It changed a shy chubby girl working as a telephone operator into a world-famous athlete, fitness writer, and gym owner—and a world-class beauty, to boot.

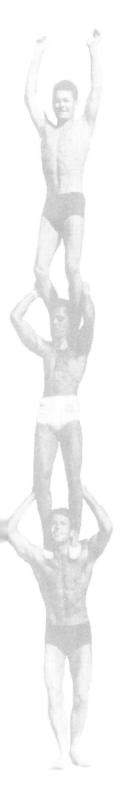

4

The Salon of Figure Development: The Gym Explosion

When Muscle Beach was founded around 1934, there were no modern "health clubs" or "spas." There were just a small number of gritty gyms for men, stocked with free weights: barbells and dumbbells. At high schools and colleges, if they had any crude weight equipment, it was only for the use of football players and wrestlers. Even then, it was kept under lock and key; too dangerous, not to mention unnatural, for anyone else to get near it. Many coaches banned weight training entirely.

"They'd say, 'you work out with weights, you're off the team,'" recalls Armand Tanny. Among the myths about weight training at that time was that it was bad for the heart, that it would cause sexual dysfunction, and that it would make a person "muscle-bound," a condition in which the joints would supposedly become hardened by an overabundance of muscle.

Weight training furthermore had unsavory and often homoerotic overtones to many people. It was a hard image to shake; it was also an easy rationalization for men who felt threatened by others with superior physiques. The stereotype was only fueled by the rise of male physique magazines in the 1940s and 1950s, which pictured nude or nearly nude men in provocative poses.

The great majority of bodybuilders, like the great majority of the population, is straight. But it's also true that some of the biggest fans of bodybuilding have always been gay. Even back in the '40s, the area a couple of miles north of Muscle Beach, known as State Beach, attracted bodybuilders . . . and gay men, who apparently liked the scenery. Today, it is common to have openly gay bodybuilders, and the gym scene among gay men is huge. In fact, many gay men complain of the pressure to beef up and be in flawless physical form, since muscle has become such an important part of the gay aesthetic.

In the early '40s, World War II would take many of the men away from the beach. Muscle Beach regulars Russ Saunders, Joe Gold, Harold Zinkin, Les Stockton, Bert Goodrich, Armand Tanny, and others served in the military. A few who had frequented Muscle Beach lost their lives or limbs in combat.

But the war years also brought new men to the beach. Hotels in the area were used as "separating centers" for servicemen preparing to go overseas. Young men from all over the country were brought to the beach area for a short period before shipping out. They may not have been in the area for long, but they got a quick education in fitness at Muscle Beach.

"They used to march down the boardwalk about six abreast, to go work out at the north side of the pier—just tons of them," recalls onetime Mr. America, wrestler, and weight lifter Armand Tanny, who was sidelined from active duty (and a chance to get

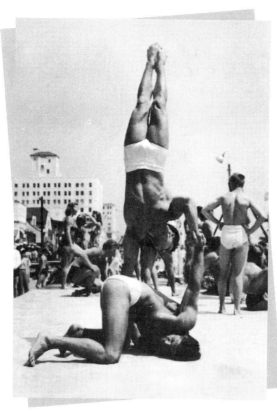

his medical degree courtesy of the federal government) by a re-
curring knee injury. "They'd see the beach action down there,
and they were just fascinated by it."

Apparently, the enlisted men liked what they saw. When the
war was over, the beach regulars returned, and many more
would flock to Southern California—and Muscle Beach. The
population of the city of Los Angeles jumped by a third from
1940 to 1950, from 1.5 million to nearly 2 million. Santa Monica's population boomed along with that of Los Angeles. By the
mid-1950s, the population of Santa Monica would reach
80,000 people. It wasn't such a small town anymore.

What's more, the war introduced countless thousands of men

to weight training and physical fitness. Men like Les Stockton and future Mr. America George Eiferman brought their weights with them to their bases and ships, and eagerly spread the word on the benefits of weight training.

More men than ever had become interested in training to build their muscles and pass the time in the military. When they came back from World War II, the popular fitness revolution went into high gear; the men were hooked, and wanted to integrate training into their new civilian lives.

There were plenty of Muscle Beach graduates poised to take advantage of this surge in interest. A number had already been in the gym business for up to a decade; it was every muscleman's dream. Gymnast Bruce Conner, Mr. America 1939 Bert Goodrich, Mr. America 1947 George Eiferman, and more than a dozen others would end up running their own gyms.

Jack LaLanne was one of the most famous. His gym was in Northern California, in Oakland. But LaLanne would often make the trip to Los Angeles and Muscle Beach to visit friends and be at the center of the burgeoning interest in fitness.

"I'd drive all day just to spend the weekend. Then a bunch of us would drive down to Long Beach [about forty miles south of Los Angeles], where there was an all-you-can-eat restaurant that charged thirty-five cents," recalled LaLanne.

LaLanne says he started experimenting with weight training at the local YMCA in Berkeley, California, when he was in his late teens. At the age of twenty-one, LaLanne abandoned earlier plans to become a doctor or chiropractor, and instead opened what he called "the nation's first modern health studio" on the third floor of an old office building in Oakland in 1936.

His rent was $45 per month when he started out. Because there was virtually no premade gym equipment at that time, except for basic barbells and dumbbells, LaLanne and others had to improvise. LaLanne enlisted the help of a machinist, who helped

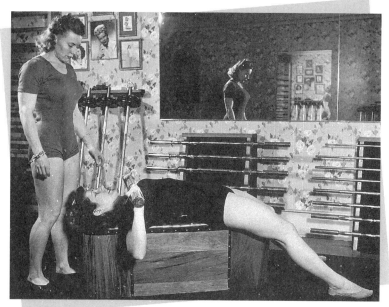

PUDGY STOCKTON TRAINING A CLIENT IN
HER GYM IN THE EARLY 1950S.

him build some rather ingenious devices. LaLanne takes credit
for developing the first leg extension machine and the first
weight selectors, among other things.

Vic Tanny was another leader in the gym business. The former schoolteacher from Rochester, New York, founded "the
first of the modern-type gyms," according to his younger brother
Armand (Vic died in the 1980s).

Vic Tanny followed his brother to Los Angeles in 1940 and
promptly founded his first gym. The genius of Vic Tanny would
be in bringing the fitness revolution of Muscle Beach, in a small
way, to thousands of people. The first of what would become
Tanny's nationwide chain of gyms opened in the loft of 1417
Second Street, in Santa Monica, just a few blocks from the pier.
There, it could draw clientele from the beach and from the
aerospace factories within a couple of miles.

"We rented that place out for $35 a month," Armand, who

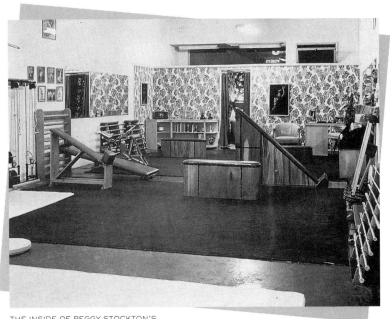

THE INSIDE OF PEGGY STOCKTON'S
GYM, ABOUT 1950.

worked with his brother in the early days, recalled. "Nobody knew anything when we first opened. People would come in and say, 'Are we supposed to pay you to lift those things?'"

The Tanny brothers would have to show visitors the ropes: what to do with the daunting combination of free weights, pulleys, and weight machines packed into the small gym. Exhibitions held in the upstairs gym attracted so many spectators that the floor was as tight as a drum. "I'm surprised the floor didn't just cave in," he said with a laugh.

Soon, people were buying enough $5-per-month memberships to allow the Tannys to tool around in a new Buick—and to fuel Vic's desire to expand. Tanny would take the one gym far beyond what anyone had done before. He quickly crossed over into the realm of "entrepreneur" (see Chapter 5).

Though their names aren't as famous as LaLanne's and Tanny's today, Pudgy and Les Stockton were highly influential in their time, too. In fact, they think they know where Tanny got the idea for the side-by-side men's and women's gyms, which he would later open—from them. Pudgy opened the quaintly named Salon of Figure Development—perhaps the first women's bodybuilding gym in the country—in 1948, on Los Angeles's famous Sunset Boulevard.

"Foremost Female Physical Culturist," boasted a promotional postcard for the gym, featuring a sepia-toned photograph of Pudgy on the beach. "Specializing in Bust Development, Figure Contouring, Reducing." Certainly the dishy photo must have prompted scores of men to pay for their wives' and girlfriends' training sessions. But Pudgy had also built up real credibility in the bodybuilding arena.

In addition to her exhibitions, she wrote on bodybuilding for women in several muscle magazines. She was a two-time "Miss Physical Culture Venus," a title bestowed by the publisher of *Physical Culture* magazine, for which she wrote a column called "Barbelles." She was even called the "female John Grimek"—a flattering comparison to the man considered to be the finest bodybuilder–weight lifter of his era.

Pudgy's gyms, like most at the time, were filled with custom-made equipment that was pretty crude by today's standards. Steel bars were attached to heavy wooden boards with bolts, then attached to pulleys to create a machine for performing "squats." Rather than the sleek, mirrors-and-neon look of later clubs, the place had a living-roomlike atmosphere, with paneling and pictures on the walls.

In 1950, Pudgy moved the gym to Beverly Hills, then opened a second location in the equally affluent community of Pasadena. In both these places, Les opened up a men's gym next door.

"Vic [Tanny] came in soon after we opened there, and said, 'Hey, this is a good idea,'" Les said. Soon after that, according to Les, Tanny began introducing side-by-side men's and women's gyms. These offered women full access to the gym while still allowing them to work out in privacy, away from prying male eyes. Other gyms, even into the early '80s, sometimes offered "women-only hours" at certain times and on certain days.

At the gym, Pudgy often put in twelve-hour days, training everyone from serious female bodybuilders to housewives. It didn't come cheaply for the time—Pudgy charged about $20 an hour for her training services—but as probably the best-known woman bodybuilder in the world, she could command that.

Other Muscle Beach folks who founded their own gyms included Bruce Conner, Walter Marcyan, George Eiferman, Bert Goodrich, George Redpath, and Karris Keirn. Most had only two or three gyms at a time, unlike Tanny with his chain of gyms,

Many of the gyms started attracting celebrities. Eiferman's gym in Las Vegas naturally got a lot of showfolk as clientele. Goodrich, Redpath, and Keirn together set up the Goodrich Gym and Health Club on Hollywood Boulevard. The gym quickly became known as "Gym to the Stars": its members included such well-known actors as James Arness and Fess Parker. Both of those actors, of course, were known for their rugged Western roles.

Women started to really take to gyms, too. Though big muscles on women wouldn't become widely accepted until the 1980s, by the '50s, female screen stars began to flaunt physiques that were obviously sculpted through exercise. The toned but still very womanly look of such stars as Jane Russell helped convince average women of the benefits of working out.

As far as competitive bodybuilding and weight lifting, though, it would be a couple of decades before a new generation of women even got back to where the women of Muscle Beach were by the 1940s and '50s. After this initial flurry of activity, women turned away from the "iron sports," associated as they

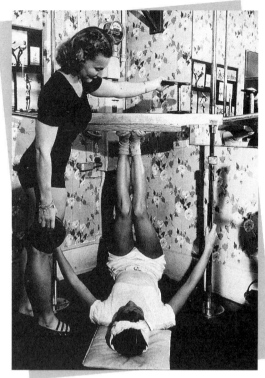

were with big, heavy men and the idea that women were becoming too "masculine."

"Women can train like horses, and they just look beautiful," says Armand Tanny. "Back then, these were very strong girls, but there were no competitions for them, so it kind of petered out after a few years."

Without a showcase and place of learning like Muscle Beach, many girls wouldn't have the opportunity to become strong, accomplished athletes. Historically, sports like weight lifting and bodybuilding became widely popular only when an energetic, dynamic backer who stood to gain something got behind them and promoted them. When a sport isn't promoted, athletes tend to lose interest or not become involved at all.

While Muscle Beach stood, the women and girls had a venue—however small. Once it was gone, though, it would take females years to regain the loss. In this sense, women lost the most when Muscle Beach closed. They lost a place to show the world that they existed.

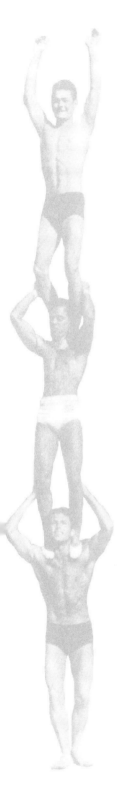

5

The Entrepreneurs

L ife's choices were simple for the denizens of Muscle Beach through the war years. They were young students, serving in the military, working odd jobs to support their modest lifestyles. Some had already opened a gym or two, the dream of nearly every Muscle Beach athlete. Beach apartments were inexpensive, and thanks to efficient public transportation, a car wasn't an absolute requirement, though most had one.

But after the war, things started to change. People were growing up, getting married, having families. Uncle Sam wasn't writing the checks anymore, and there was a housing squeeze. It was time to find a way to make a real living.

Opening a gym, especially as rents climbed, could prove expensive and difficult. It often meant long days and little freedom to take time off. It's not surprising, then, that those who saw the enormous moneymaking potential in fitness, especially with the spread of mass communication through television, decided to find an alternative route, becoming "muscle capitalists."

There had been muscle capitalists before, entrepreneurs with a knack for marketing, myth-making, and boosterism. There was turn-of-the-century strongman Eugen Sandow, who became internationally famous through his exhibitions and lent his name to a variety of fitness products. A little later, former "97-pound weakling" Charles Atlas—born Angelo Siciliano, and raised in New York—created a lucrative mail-order operation with his "dynamic tension" training method. These two muscle merchants actually discouraged weight training, since it wasn't in their economic interests. It took decades to reverse popular misconceptions put forth by such influential salesmen.

Bob Hoffman created York Barbell, and later a line of diet supplements, as a side operation to his money-making oil-burner factory. By the start of World War II, he was making a healthy living with these businesses, in addition to their primary promotional tool, his *Strength & Health* magazine. The Weiders would later build a similar empire with their bodybuilding magazines, vitamins, and supplements.

As the benefits of weight training became more widely accepted and as gym membership rose to include tens of thousands of "normal" people—businessmen and housewives, not just "muscleheads"—there was a clear opportunity to capitalize on the trend. Owning a gym was a hard way to make a living, requiring constant work, upkeep, and expenditures of cash to do it right.

Creating one hit product, on the other hand, could pay off for years. Although it's always difficult to come up with a great idea that is both practical and popular, if one can do it, the product can turn into a steady earner with relatively little further outlay of cash.

History shows that it's often not the first person who invents something who gets the glory. Rather, it's the person who has the resources and smarts to figure out how to market his invention on a mass scale. Such was the case with those who developed and marketed various exercise machines.

Muscle Beach regular Harold Zinkin is credited with bringing out the Universal machine. Like many others, Zinkin, a fine all-around athlete (a gymnast and a bodybuilder) and World War II veteran, had opened a gym after the war. But it was his exercise machine that became a cash cow and ended up making him wealthier than most of his Muscle Beach brethren.

Others had been jerry-rigging machines for years, out of iron, wood, and pulley systems. People built on the clever ideas of others, striving to come up with the next tweak or twist that would make their machine unique.

A machinist helped custom-make innovative, attractive, and functional equipment for Jack LaLanne's early gyms. But it was Zinkin who put it all together in a ready-made, compact, marketable exercise machine on which you could perform many different exercises.

The development of weight machines would prove a strong selling point for people who were intimidated by working out with free weights. The self-contained style of the machines also made them popular for institutional use. Those who did any weight training in school during the '60s and '70s probably were introduced to the Universal machine.

The design itself was strikingly simple, yet ingenious: a set of benches and pulleys built around a central frame on which weights were loaded. The device became so popular that it became the model for many later gym-quality machines, in addition to systems that were later widely sold for home use.

Another popular weight system was marketed by Walter Marcyan, also a Muscle Beach regular and onetime gym owner.

Like many at the beach who shortened or Americanized their names for show business or simply for the sake of fitting in, Marcyan went by Marcy. That's what he called his gym system: the Marcy Gym.

As is the case with many young businesses, companies like these would end up fighting each other from time to time in court over who invented what when, and who held the patent on particular machine features. A slightly different pulley system or design feature can make all the difference when it comes to cases of alleged patent infringement.

It's a testament to the popularity of both the Universal and Marcy machines, though, that both names are still around today. Other companies have come and gone. Others may have taken the lead today in state-of-the-art gym equipment, but these two brands remain widely recognized.

Jack LaLanne also found numerous ways to capitalize on his growing fame as a fitness icon. LaLanne would license his name for use on everything from a chain of health clubs owned by Bally Corporation to nutritional supplements and home-exercise equipment. Probably his greatest contribution, though, was his 1950s television show. It was through TV that he was able to reach the greatest number of people, and to use his genius for gab and motivation.

Then there was Vic Tanny, considered by many to be the father of the modern gym chain. After opening his first gym near the beach in Santa Monica, Tanny quickly saw the potential to launch a whole chain of gyms rather than just a single location. Other Muscle Beachers had opened two or three, even a handful. But it was Tanny who would open dozens, nationwide.

Tanny opened two more gyms around L.A. in the early 1940s: one just a little further north and east in Santa Monica, and another on Wilshire Boulevard in L.A.'s toney Miracle Mile shopping district. He briefly opened one in the Belmont shore

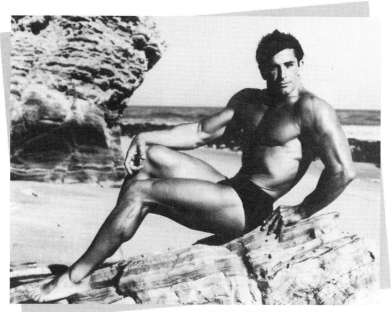

ARMAND TANNY IN A PROMOTIONAL SHOT.

area of Long Beach (a coastal town just south of greater Los Angeles) in 1941. It was right near the Belmont Pier.

But the attack on Pearl Harbor brought a quick end to that gym: fearful of the West Coast being attacked by Japan, the government made citizens and businesses alike cover their windows and turn off lights at night. Also, it became difficult to acquire gym equipment once the war was on.

By the war's end, Tanny had several children to support. He was itching to finally expand. His equation was a simple one: more gyms equaled more people equaled more money. Sign people up to contracts, and you have a guaranteed revenue stream that you can bring to the bank and borrow money against. Use the money to open even more gyms. Repeat the process over and over again, ad infinitum.

Tanny's brainstorm came around the time that retail chains of various sorts were just beginning to take hold in the United States. Soon, supermarkets, retail stores, restaurants, and other businesses once run as mom-and-pop operations would be controlled largely by big corporations. Why not fitness shops? The business could benefit from the economies of scale, and people would favor a fancy, brand-name gym over a no-name one.

Tanny was absolutely right, to a point. His expansion was rapid: by the early 1950s, he owned and operated a total of forty-four gyms around Southern California. Their red carpeting and gleaming chrome machines attracted folks who would never have stepped inside a dank weight-lifting gym, and by 1960 he'd expanded to the East Coast and was spending a reported $2 million a year on advertising alone.

"[Vic Tanny] did what they call taking the gyms out of the cellar," says Tanny's brother and onetime business partner, Armand. "They were beautiful little places. One gym even had all gold-plated equipment."

Tanny gyms began offering either separate men's and women's facilities, or alternate hours and days for women. Though women were becoming more interested in going to the gym as a way to "reduce," many still weren't comfortable sweating alongside men who might ogle them, hit on them, or worse, find them unfeminine because they were working out with weights.

The variety of offerings of these gyms followed the popular fashions of the times. Saunas and whirlpools were added to give more of the "spa" atmosphere desired by female patrons. Now-laughable machines, such as one on which a person (usually female) stood and let a motorized belt do the "exercise," were added in droves. Just because people became interested in going to gyms didn't mean they actually wanted to work hard. But most of the equipment was sound.

By the early '60s, there were eighty-four Vic Tanny gyms in the United States. There were an estimated 300,000 members. But, in a common business tale of too much, too fast, Tanny's empire started to crumble.

Tanny first started to get into trouble for his employees' hard-ball business tactics. Tanny and his salesmen were notoriously hard sellers: a Tanny salesman in Chicago was accused of false imprisonment, for allegedly not letting a woman leave his office for an hour while he tried to get her to sign a contract. The press wasn't exactly good when this kind of news was leaked.

Tanny himself was said to have distributed a memo to the sales staff of his gyms, with suggested phone pitches to prospective customers. It ran through every technique imaginable to break down the resistance of potential members, and get them to come in for an appointment. At the bottom of the memo, salesmen were told: "If you fail to get an appointment, then take a gun out of the desk and shoot yourself."

But these kinds of reports weren't the worst of it for Tanny. In the summer of 1962, five finance companies seized Tanny's New York clubs when he ran out of money. On paper, he'd sold $9 million worth of new memberships in the New York area. However, many of the new members who had responded to Tanny's ad blitz and high-pressure sales tactics defaulted on their payments, shutting off the cash flow that Tanny had counted on.

It was the five finance companies that then closed half of the Tanny gyms in New York. These companies took the Tanny name off some of the remaining clubs and refused to honor previously sold Tanny memberships. The memberships hadn't been cheap: some had paid up to $395 for a three-year membership—a sizable sum in 1962. The whole affair was an embarrassment to Tanny and left a sour taste in many people's mouths about the health-club business. The whole industry became suspect for high-pressure sales tactics and for running fly-by-night operations.

Still, Tanny was able to continue capitalizing on his name. Even in the wake of the gym closings, Tanny came out with a Vic Tanny Home Gym, a line of health foods, and other products. He never achieved his dream, though, of rebuilding his gym empire and of having "10 million Americans working out in the Vic Tanny system," as he'd told *Newsweek* magazine in 1963. Tanny died in the early 1980s in Florida, where he lived in the last years of his life.

Armand Tanny, younger than Vic by about eight years and a more accomplished athlete—he was Mr. America 1950 and an Olympic-caliber weight lifter—had left the Tanny gym business long before it ran aground in the 1960s. He became a longtime editor and writer for the Weider publication *Muscle and Fitness.*

Armand's daughter, Mandy, has kept the Tanny name alive in the fitness business. She, too, writes for *Muscle and Fitness,* has written books on sports nutrition, and has her own gym in Woodland Hills, California: Tanny's Personal Fitness.

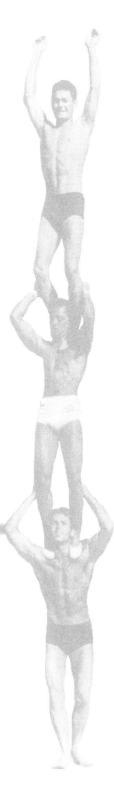

6

The Performers

Everyone was a performer at Muscle Beach. Even in the earliest days of a simple mat on the sand, scores of people would crowd around for the chance to see the remarkable stunts. As the years went on, it became a huge event. Weekends, particularly holidays, were a nonstop show, with up to three or four thousand spectators jammed into the area.

Many Muscle Beachers would also be asked to go to nearby private beach clubs, like the swanky Del Mar Club, to put on gymnastics and diving shows for members. Though they were ostensibly performing free of charge, many of the young athletes didn't turn it down if they were offered some cash by their appreciative fans.

Muscle Beach had always had a connection to professional performers of stage and screen. In addition to the pros who would drop by to par-

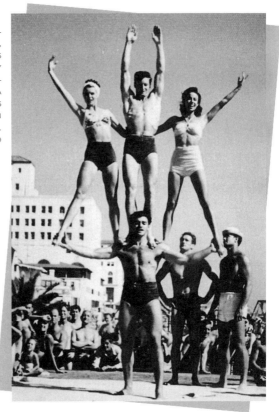

ticipate in the activities, many of the locals were famous, too. The stretch of Santa Monica Beach beginning just north of the pier and winding up the coast was well known as a playground for the rich and famous. Such stars as Mae West, Douglas Fairbanks, and Cary Grant had swank beach "cottages" to the north of the Santa Monica Pier. The area became known as the Gold Coast, an early version of today's star-studded Malibu beachfront scene.

After World War II, the beach became only more popular. It also really started to live up to its name: it became all about muscle. The popularity of weight lifting was rising fast, and the sport of bodybuilding was beginning to take hold. The first Mr.

America contest had been held just before the war, in 1939. Bert Goodrich was the winner, becoming the first of many early Mr. Americas to grace Santa Monica's beach on a regular basis.

Goodrich, an ex-circus performer, became a chief petty officer in charge of physical training instruction. While in the service, he met several of the men with whom he would become associated at the beach, including gymnast and future gym partner George Redpath. During this time, Goodrich also met Norma Tanny, sister of Vic and Armand. The two were married, linking two of the "royal families" of Muscle Beach.

Weights were given greater emphasis on the Muscle Beach platform starting around 1948. There had always been some weights there, brought by the performers and used in a small area near the equipment shack abutting the platform. But now they were becoming a main attraction, taking up a larger part of the platform. Barone Leone, a wrestler with long flowing hair who lived near the beach and was a frequent judge of the physique contests there, is said to have donated the first major, permanent collection of weights to Muscle Beach in the late 1940s.

Along with these beefy, tanned bodybuilders came some stunning women, too. Screen bombshell Jayne Mansfield, who married a bodybuilder (European transplant Mickey Hargitay), would sometimes visit Muscle Beach. Actress Jane Russell was also a somewhat frequent visitor.

Russell had a very specific reason for her keen interest in Muscle Beach: she had her eye on Bob Waterfield, a football star who frequently played volleyball there, near the Muscle Beach platform. "She would come down looking for him. She would hound him, and they finally did get married. . . . Boy, she really pursued him," recalled one of the Muscle Beach ladies who was there at the time.

As the fame of Muscle Beach's bodybuilders grew, entertainer Mae West even drew from the talent there to appear in her sold-out, nationally touring live revue in 1954. Mickey Hargitay, Joe Gold, who later founded Gold's Gym and World Gym, and Armand Tanny were among those chosen for West's beefcake brigade. This, of course, was decades before Madonna surrounded herself with oiled-up, well-muscled men.

The meeting between West and the musclemen took place at her rather rococo white-and-gold-decorated apartment in Hollywood's Ravenswood Building. The get-together was arranged by former Mr. America and Muscle Beach regular George Eiferman, who'd been introduced to and become friends with West several years before. The whole idea for the show came out of conversations between Eiferman and West, who was a well-known connoisseur of the male form.

In her 1959 autobiography, *Goodness Had Nothing to Do with It,* West recalled being introduced to some of the men who would become her beefy backups. Well past her prime as one of the screen's first sex symbols—but still as lusty and busty as ever—West was sixty-two at the time of the meeting. "They arrived, their suits bursting with health, and my butler ushered them into my living room. There were only a dozen, but the room looked crowded," recalled West cheekily.

When she launched her nightclub act in 1954, West hadn't been seen onscreen for eleven years. Her career had taken a dive partly due to the restrictions that were placed on her following the passage of the morality-policing film production code (aka the Hays Code). After a few disappointing movies that had her playing cleaned-up characters, West had all but disappeared from the spotlight.

But West's enduring fame, as well as the novel appeal of a stage full of musclemen, attracted record crowds wherever they toured around the country for three years, starting at the Sahara Club in Las Vegas.

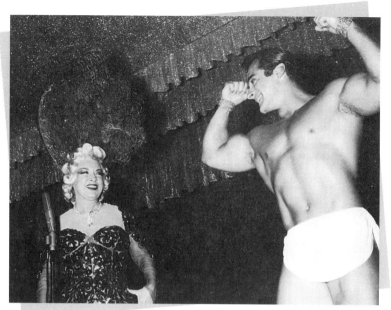

MAE WEST AND GEORGE EIFERMAN IN HER
HIT STAGE REVUE.

Tanny recalled the show fondly. "Mae had her traditional set-tee there. She'd be laying there with her big boobs hanging out, watching us as we came out one by one in our robes. . . . We'd come out and stand there with our backs to the audience, then open our robes. And she'd open her mouth and act ecstatic. No-body knew whether we had anything on underneath," Tanny said with a laugh.

Later in the show, the men strutted their stuff wearing only small, toga-style briefs and sandals. The combination of brawn and West's incomparably ribald humor made for sell-out crowds wherever the show went. Both Tanny and Eiferman recall the tour as a record-breaker in terms of the box-office receipts. Tanny also recalls that West had strict standards for her support-ing cast, even offstage: the men were to dress in suits and ties when accompanying Ms. West to dinner in the evenings. It was all part of the carefully cultivated image that made West an icon.

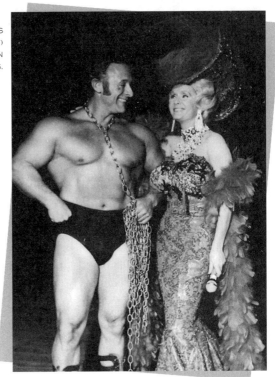

West also hoped that a number of her musclemen would go on to successful careers in show business after the tour was over. That didn't really materialize. Outside of bit parts for a number of the men, Hargitay probably came closest, through his marriage to Mansfield.

Hollywood may not have known what to do with them, but the boys were sure a hit with the ladies, both onstage and off. Though they don't brag about it today, the rumor is they never had reason to be plagued with the fabled "loneliness of the road."

Eiferman always had a puppy-eyed, boyish charm about him that was only accentuated by his musculature. Armand Tanny, by contrast, was the prototypical he-man, deeply tanned and slightly dangerous looking. The men who were Muscle Beach regulars sometimes joke that if they're the last one left standing, they'll write the book about all of their exploits. But that's not likely to happen, since these rogues share a code of honor and discretion among themselves.

West's nightclub act was so popular that, years later in 1970, Debbie Reynolds would pay homage to it in her own Vegas stage show. Eiferman was then in his mid-forties and the owner of a gym in Las Vegas that was popular with celebrities and regular casino workers alike. He reprised his role as a toga-wearing muscleman alongside Reynolds, who was dressed up in a wig and elaborate costume to look like West.

One of the beefy men who joined West on her tour was Chuck Krauser, a friend of Gold's from the merchant marine. Krauser was a former wrestler and circus roustabout, a little rough around the edges like most of the guys on the tour. None of them were born with silver spoons in their mouths.

But a funny thing happened that was straight out of a Hollywood movie: Krauser and West hit it off. Thirty years her junior, Krauser was instantly smitten with the indomitable and still-striking West. It was an unlikely love story, but then, nothing about West was ever typical. The two quickly became inseparable.

At her suggestion, he soon changed his name to the more classy-sounding Paul Novak. It was actually the second name change for the sometime-wrestler and circus roustabout: he was born Chester Ribonsky in Baltimore and changed his name to Krauser because he thought it a more fitting name for a wrestler.

In any case, the couple remained committed to each other, though unmarried, until West's death in 1980 at the age of eighty-seven. Friends credit Krauser with helping West to lead a

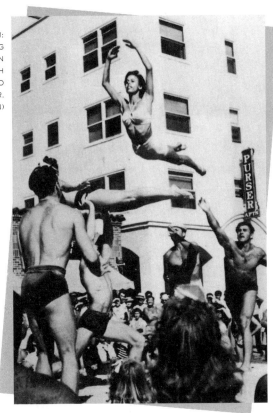

ON THE PLATFORM:
PAULA BOELSEMS BEING
TOSSED BY AL JACKSON
AND RAN HALL, WITH
RUSS SAUNDERS POISED
TO CATCH HER.
(CARL R. NIELSON)

comfortable life at home up until the end. Krauser nursed her in her final days and lived another nineteen years himself. He passed away in July 1999 in Santa Monica, at the age of seventy-six.

The week before he died, Krauser, who was weakened by prostate cancer but alert, reflected on his remarkable life story. Surrounded by such longtime friends as Joe Gold, he was said to have summed it all up simply: "I've had such a great, incredible life."

The stage wasn't the only place for the population of Muscle Beach to find work in show business. Movies offered another natural outlet. Though only Steve Reeves would go on to top-billed movie stardom, many others stayed busy with bit parts and stunt work in films. Hollywood could always use a man who was strong, handsome, and fearless.

Muscle Beach's most successful stuntman, and one of its guiding lights over the decades, was Russ Saunders. The wiry native of rural western Canada taught himself gutsy, often daredevil stunts while playing with his seven siblings as a child. Smitten with acrobatics and show biz at a young age, he volunteered to carry water for the circus when it was in town just to be close to the action.

It's no surprise, then, that Saunders took to California immediately upon his first visit, and never left. "The weather was perfect for someone who loved being outdoors, and there was so much going on here," recalled Saunders. He quickly found Muscle Beach, and over the years, his siblings and mother would also become visitors there.

With his athletic ability and slim good looks, Saunders soon got work as a stuntman, doubling for such stars as Douglas Fairbanks and Gene Kelly over the years. He was a top stuntman for decades.

Saunders had more of a dancer's body than a bodybuilder's. Though he was also expert at diving, balancing, and tumbling, his specialty at the beach was adagio—a graceful form of dance-like acrobatics performed by two people (usually, a man tossing and catching a female partner). Paula Unger became his longtime partner; she too would become a stunt performer in many films.

Saunders's stunt work led to other things as well. One day while on contract to Warner Bros., he was called into the office of Jack Warner. He was slightly apprehensive about why the big boss would want to see him but reported to the executive offices dutifully.

It turned out that legendary artist Salvador Dalí was there, looking for a model to represent Jesus in his famous painting "Christ of St. John of the Cross." After looking over Saunders in his tights, Dalí chose Saunders as his model. Posing for the artist became one of Saunders's proudest accomplishments.

The license plate on Saunders's modest Toyota today reads DALI2, and he delights in showing people photocopies of the painting and of the inscription Dalí wrote to him in a book of his work. Like many people who work in Hollywood, Saunders seems to regard movies as work, and "real" art as a higher form of expression.

Saunders would eventually work on more than 500 films. He was usually totally unrecognizable in his roles, but he and Paula would occasionally get to perform some acrobatics on-camera, as in a sequence in *Thoroughly Modern Millie* with Carol Channing. He worked for more than a dozen years with TV's *Circus of the Stars,* teaching celebrities tumbling and teeterboard tricks. He would continue to do stunt work through the 1980s.

Even though his movie work kept him extremely busy, Saunders would come to Muscle Beach every weekend to put on shows and to teach others. He recalled his distinctive opening act: "I'd park my car in the lot next to the beach, run up and do a flip over the benches," Saunders said, circling his hand in the air, "and grab the hat off a man on my way if he happened to be sitting there."

Saunders married a fellow acrobat, Patti Bivens Taylor; the couple and their son became one of the beach's most prominent families. Over the years, Saunders nurtured thousands of young athletes, some of whom went on to become Olympic or professional competitors, or coaches.

After a long career performing together on the beach, in exhibitions and in filmed entertainment, Saunders and Paula Unger Boelsems became the United States's first accredited judges for the International Federation of Sports Acrobatics.

They traveled the world, from North America to Asia to Africa, teaching clinics and judging meets in the new competitive sport.

Though most of these Muscle Beach alumni aren't household names, their influence was great. They took the traditional path for people to learn about fitness—friend to friend, relative to relative, word of mouth—and exploded it into a national phenomenon. Time and again, it's true that entertainment can be a powerful medium not just to amuse, but also to teach.

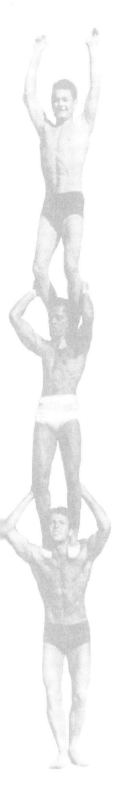

7

Teachers and Students

Over the years, many professional athletes and actors would visit the beach. One of the most illustrious was Babe Didrikson, who won two track and field medals at the 1932 Olympics and was still considered one of the very finest all-around female athletes in history. She married professional wrestler George Zaharias, who also was a frequent visitor at the beach. The couple are remembered by Muscle Beach alumni as nice, down-to-earth people in spite of their fame.

Another top female athlete, skater Sonja Henie, became associated with Muscle Beach when she came to L.A. in the summer of 1936 to make her first professional appearance at the L.A. Coliseum. The talented and photogenic Henie was a medalist in three Olympics—1928, 1932, and 1936. Immediately after her win in 1936, she was courted by Fox studios to become a film star.

Henie's move to Hollywood meant work for a number of local skaters. One of these was Gene Thesloff (who later changed his name to Tesloff—it drove him crazy when people pronounced the silent *h*), an East Coast transplant who had been learning some tricks at Muscle Beach. An amateur when he arrived, he was fairly athletic and had done a good deal of skating. But he was raw material and certainly wasn't making a living at it. In fact, he paid the bills by working as a ticket taker at Grauman's Chinese Theater on Hollywood Boulevard, one of the premier movie houses of the era.

Muscle Beach colleague Ran Hall recalled Thesloff upon his arrival at the beach as "a big guy and quite awkward, but . . . strong." Soon, Thesloff was practicing handstands, and tossing and balancing the more experienced athletes at Muscle Beach. His increased grace and agility paid off: Thesloff tried out for and gained a part in Henie's first movie, *Thin Ice,* which was a typical "lovely commoner girl attracts dashing prince" yarn. He went on to appear in several other Henie pictures after that, and then launched his own solo skating career.

Working with Henie, Thesloff met Ann Taylor, a young skater who was picked from the Los Angeles Figure Skating Club to appear in Henie's film. Thesloff and Taylor became a star act in their own right, headlining shows all over the country. The pair wowed audiences with their innovative acrobatic moves. According to Hall, Thesloff and Taylor were the first to perform high-lift adagio, a form of acrobatics popular with the Muscle Beach crowd, on ice. These moves are now an integral part of figure-skating routines today.

Thesloff later married a pretty Swedish skating champion, Vivi Ann Hulten. The couple were frequent visitors to Muscle Beach until they moved to Minneapolis. There, they became top figure-skating instructors for years, until Thesloff's death.

Of course, there were many other professional athletes who

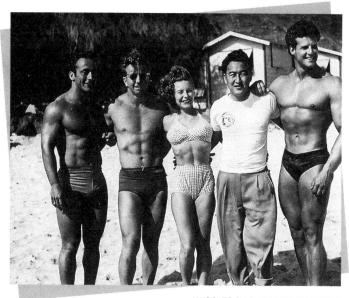

MUSCLES ON THE BEACH IN HAWAII:
(FROM LEFT) GEORGE EIFERMAN, LES
AND PUDGY STOCKTON, AN UNIDEN-
TIFIED HAWAIIAN MAN, AND STEVE
REEVES.

passed through Muscle Beach more fleetingly over the years. George Eiferman recalls such varied sports stars as race-car driver Greg Breedlove and champion golfer Frank Stranahan visiting Muscle Beach in the 1940s.

Muscle Beach produced and hosted many bodybuilding title-holders, including first Mr. America Bert Goodrich, George Eiferman, and Steve Reeves. These titles were great honors and produced terrific opportunities for these men to do tours or perform in movies. But bodybuilding wasn't (and still isn't, despite great efforts by Joe Weider and others) an Olympic sport. In a testament to the egalitarian opportunities at the beach, Muscle Beach's most famous Olympian was a woman: diver Pat McCormick.

McCormick won Gold medals at both the 1952 and 1956 games. She got her early training at the beach from Muscle

Beach fixture and women's exercise proponent Barney Fry, who taught her swimming, diving, and martial arts moves. In 1957 Fry crowed to the *Saturday Evening Post:* "When she was only twelve years old she could lift four hundred and ninety pounds and do thirty-five push-ups. And she used to wrestle and throw guys that weighed two hundred pounds. In those days she weighed only ninety pounds herself."

Some of those at Muscle Beach, like Fry, ended up discovering a knack for encouraging and teaching others. Such was the case with George Eiferman, the Mr. America from Philadelphia who helped Mae West assemble the musclemen for her famous 1950s stage show. The affable Eiferman lectured on fitness at schools around the country for years. With a 100-pound dumbbell in one hand and a trumpet in the other, he took his show on the road to literally thousands of schools. The former Mr. America, Mr. Universe, and amateur musician dedicated himself, even while he was running gyms and starting a family, to spreading the word that "working out with weights can change your life."

Eiferman's is the quintessential tale of a 97-pound-weakling-turned-Adonis. Like many early musclemen, he was the scrawny child of immigrant parents—his father was Hungarian, his mother Russian. He grew up in a tough neighborhood in Philadelphia, "the skinniest kid in the neighborhood. I got beat up by bullies," he said. Eiferman's physical disadvantage had begun at birth: he was born prematurely and weighed less than five pounds when he was born. He was always small for his age.

America entered the war, and Eiferman joined the navy at age seventeen. By that time, his interest had already become piqued about weight training. Philadelphia wasn't far from the town of York, Pennsylvania, where Bob Hoffman had built up his York Barbell compound. Eiferman got hooked when he saw what the York guys were doing.

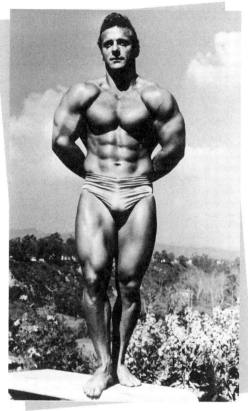

Before reporting for duty, Eiferman bought himself a set of weights. He brought them onto the ship with him and started training and teaching others on board. "The guys really took to it; it gave them something to do," Eiferman recalls.

Probably none of his navy colleagues had more success than young Eiferman himself, though, at effecting a dramatic change in his body through weight training. When he returned home from the war four years later, Eiferman's family barely recognized him: he'd gone from 135 pounds to 190. The gain was pure muscle, packed solidly onto his five-foot-seven frame.

Despite his impressive physical achievement, Eiferman didn't immediately decide to devote himself to becoming a bodybuilder. He figured he'd return to his first love, music. Body-building for him was a very intense pursuit, but still a hobby. He attended the Philadelphia Music Academy, studying trumpet. His dream was to be in a big band.

Eiferman made a go of it for a couple of years. He taught instrumental music in the public schools, and put together a small group to play at dances and other local events. They got steady work but were nothing remarkable. Soon enough, it became clear that he wasn't going to become a top horn player for a band like Glenn Miller's or Tommy Dorsey's. Eiferman had a burning desire to do something where he could make it to the top.

He decided to try to actively pursue bodybuilding, something at which he'd already had proven success. He entered and won the Mr. Philadelphia physique contest in 1947, a remarkable feat for the skinny kid who'd been a target for bullies just a dozen years before. He experienced the sweet taste of success that he'd never gotten with his musical pursuits, where he'd always been just another horn player.

The next step and ultimate goal at that point for Eiferman was getting to Santa Monica's Muscle Beach, which by then was world famous. "It was the mecca," Eiferman said simply. It's where he felt he needed to be.

But it was a big move. Housing in California was scarce in the postwar years, and Eiferman had little money. Many men would have resigned themselves to staying and making the best of it in Philly. Not Eiferman. Determined to find a way to get to Muscle Beach, he sat down and wrote a letter to Vic Tanny, who by then was a well-known gym owner.

He practically begged Tanny to give him a place to sleep in exchange for his training services. Tanny agreed; Eiferman says he slept on the trampoline in Tanny's Santa Monica gym for months after landing in Santa Monica in 1947, until he could afford an apartment.

Eiferman trained customers at Tanny's gym to earn his keep. Meanwhile, he set his sights on the Mr. America title: he placed fifth in '47. He was disappointed, but again, he redoubled his efforts rather than throwing in the towel. After a year of intense training, he won the title in 1948; he would also become Mr. Universe, one of the professional titles that was quickly being added to the stable of possible honors for bodybuilders.

What followed was a somewhat typical career trajectory for a star of Muscle Beach: Eiferman ended up opening gyms in Las Vegas and Hawaii. In the late '40s, he toured with some Muscle Beach colleagues, including Steve Reeves and Les and Pudgy Stockton, putting on strength and bodybuilding exhibitions. And, of course, he helped organize and took part in the wildly successful Mae West show in the '50s.

Eiferman was a bit of a clown, someone who didn't take himself too seriously and put his charm, humor, and good looks to work for him. He would sometimes insert jokes and pratfalls into his routines to develop rapport with an audience that otherwise might have been in awe of, or even resentful of, such a fine-looking specimen of masculinity. He wasn't afraid to fall down or dress in drag for a laugh.

But on the serious side, Eiferman became a thirty-year spokesman for fitness in the public schools. The year he won the Mr. America competition, the head of an organization that provided school assembly speakers across the United States approached Eiferman about taking his one-man musical/muscular show on the road. Eiferman agreed, considering it an honor to be able to teach, and a way of giving back some of the goodwill he'd received over the last couple of years.

Combining the humor of a clown, the physique of a bodybuilder, and the talent of a musician, Eiferman was a unique motivational speaker. For forty-five minutes, he entertained and taught by doing his simultaneous trumpet playing/barbell-lifting gag, easily hoisting the heaviest kids in school into the air and lecturing earnestly on the benefits of fitness. He helped bridge the gap between musicians, often thought of as nerdy, and the athletic jocks; he got compliments from both band teachers and sports coaches.

For years, Eiferman handed out small, printed cards bearing his picture and philosophy. These "Ten Daily Exercises" were listed on the inside of the folded card:

1. A good eye exercise—See also the perfection in others. See the everlasting beauty in human kindness.
2. A good tongue exercise—Speak from the heart instead of the mouth.
3. A good facial exercise—A smile often repeated.
4. Hearing exercise—When we speak we learn nothing. Listening is the teacher. Then speak.
5. Brain exercise—Think only constructive thoughts. Good reading is to the mind what exercise is to the body.
6. Leg exercise—Walk toward knowledge, wisdom, health, and brotherhood of all men.
7. Breathing exercise—Inhale the great works of music, art, literature, and philosophy. Exhale spitefulness and other negative thoughts.
8. Strength exercise—Have the strength to endure when things are unendurable, to pass the next test after failing the recent one.
9. Heart exercise—Have the heart to "Constructively" improve Self, our Environment, Community, and Country.
10. Soul exercise—We are never alone. Walk with God.

Alongside these "exercises" were printed a few additional kernels of philosophy. "Probably the greatest discovery anyone can make is that we can change our life for the better, by changing our immature, negative attitude to MATURE, constructive attitudes," it read. The type of mind-over-body philosophy has always been popular with speakers and writers on fitness. Jack LaLanne preached it; in muscle magazine articles decades later, Arnold Schwarzenegger would also extol the mental aspect of training.

Other bodybuilders, like Armand Tanny, downplay the importance of this type of mental/emotional component to training. They say it's purely about the physical, not the mental. But others will say that this approach inspired them and helped them in other walks of life.

Eiferman, for one, always considered his school presentations one of his proudest achievements. In all, he visited more than 5,000 schools over three decades. Though teaching wasn't his profession, it turned out to be a calling for him.

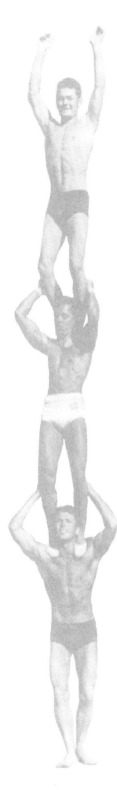

8
The Nature Boys

That's what they called them: Nature Boys. They were a group of men who lived outdoors, ate organic foods plucked straight from the ground or tree, and were scruffy in appearance.

Today, you can see their spiritual counterparts taking yoga classes, getting smeared with seaweed and mud at fancy spas, buying New Age books, and shopping for tofu and organic vegetables at the thousands of health-food stores around the country. It's no longer considered bizarre to want to commune with nature and eat natural foods.

But in mid-century America, these men were called a variety of names... "fruitcakes" and "wackos," for example. In later years, these free spirits would be called other things: beatniks, hippies, maybe even bums. But in the 1940s, this curious native California species of "health nut" would become part of the Muscle Beach landscape.

Long-haired, wild-eyed, and bearded, the Nature Boys were worlds apart from the clean-cut athletes of Muscle Beach. They wore beads and sandals instead of work-out trunks; they were tan and trim, but the acrobats' daily physical routines were too regimented for them. What the two groups had in common was their interest in health foods, healthy living, and putting on a show. The Nature Boys became a colorful part of the Muscle Beach scene starting in the early 1940s.

They were the "original hippies," boasts Gypsy Boots (real name Robert Bootzin), apparently the last of the Nature Boys still around—and in remarkably good health at the age of ninety. In many ways, they did live the prototypical hippie life, living off the land and espousing peace and love among all people.

They promoted natural foods—mostly fresh, raw vegetables, nuts and fruits, which they gathered locally—and a back-to-nature lifestyle. In fact, the seeds of the natural/organic foods movement, which most of us associate with the 1960s and 1970s, actually came from the Nature Boys and their followers. The fact that they were in California—where so many trends originate, and where they rubbed shoulders with well-known athletes and celebrities—helped speed their message to the mainstream.

Today, there are hundreds of private stores, co-ops, and even chains of shops specializing in "whole" foods. Farmer's markets have become very popular places for city dwellers to find fresh vegetables. Mainstream supermarkets devote sections to organic foods, and drugstores carry aisles of "natural" supplements.

Back in the '40s and '50s, the Nature Boys came to the beach to preach their philosophy to the crowds, sell fruits and nuts to the acrobats and bodybuilders, and add some general levity to the proceedings. They made music, cracked jokes, and generally played the part of court jesters at Muscle Beach.

The ragtag bunch went by names such as Gypsy Gene (he never revealed his given name), Fred Bushnoff—a character known in his native San Francisco as the "Mayor of Russian Hill"—and Gypsy Boots, also sometimes known as Figaro, after a loopy version of "Figaro" he would sing while picking figs. Before everyone came to know them as Nature Boys, more conventional folks would jokingly call these three "the Smith brothers," after the bearded men depicted on the cough-drop tins. Beards weren't exactly the rage in the 1940s, so the three stood out all the more.

There was also Bob Wallace, a Nature Boy commonly known as Jesus. Why? "He looked just like Jesus—the right coloring, the long dark hair, and he always wore a robe and sandals," explains Pudgy Stockton. Wallace played up the resemblance. Unlike most of the Nature Boys, who tended to mix a bit of Eastern philosophy with a laid-back, live-and-let-live attitude, he went beyond preaching health. "Jesus" preached his own view of the Gospel, using the beach as his soapbox.

Muscle Beach regulars recall that the Nature Boys provided an offbeat contrast at the beach. Pudgy Stockton says: "I can't remember which one it was, but one [of the Nature Boys] would get up at the beach, when there were a lot of people around, and would hold up a big bunch of carrots that looked like they'd just been pulled from the ground. Then he'd go into this big speech about eating raw vegetables. . . ."

Les Stockton piped in, "But he'd lose his audience when he started talking about the horse manure he'd spread all over his body! Oh boy, everyone's listening, then he has to throw in something like that," said Stockton with a laugh, reminiscing about some of the nuttier "natural" things the Nature Boys were into.

The Nature Boys extolled the virtues of raw food years before "natural foods" proponents like Euell Gibbons became widely famous. They exercised for health but were not into muscle-building and athletics so much as they were into an overall "natural" lifestyle. That meant living for periods of time in the canyons around Southern California, sleeping on the beach, and generally finding ways to keep from having to put on a suit and tie and go to an office.

One of Boots's best-known stunts at the beach involved his ability to throw a football enormous distances: fifty or sixty yards, he says, from the Muscle Beach platform toward the ocean. "Whenever I went to the beach," he recalls, "I'd carry a football, a tambourine, and a basket of fruit."

He was also known for his comedy routines. He was always playing the jester, letting himself be tossed around by wrestlers on the platform, or dressing up in a clown outfit to perform stunts. He was fearless and limber, if not as graceful as the acrobats. And if being part of the Muscle Beach action was what got people to notice you, Boots was there. Like some of the beach's most famous athletes, he had a nose for showmanship and self-promotion.

The Nature Boys were very visible at the beach, but their area of influence was much wider. In his 1993 self-published autobiography *The Gypsy in Me!*, Boots—the son of Russian immigrants—describes the Nature Boys as "a merry band of bearded, mop-haired, half-naked vegetarians who wandered around in the hills, occasionally rolling into town like a pack of wild men . . . we had a common desire to abandon civilization and to live a natural, healthy life."

They roamed from the desert east of Los Angeles, around Palm Springs, to the rugged canyons of Los Angeles and down to the beach. Though expert at avoiding traditional nine-to-five work, many of the Nature Boys had enough musical, literary, or just plain "schmoozing" talent to sustain themselves and to continue living their quirky lives. Boots worked on a farm part of the time, where he could be outdoors, make some money, and have fresh food to sell.

The lifestyle seemed to include liberal amounts of women and song, if not wine (that wasn't part of the diet regimen and was considered detrimental to overall health). But like the exercise crusaders, they knew sex was a key motivator. In addition to touting the "cleansing" and healthful effects of foods such as sprouts and figs, they espoused the aphrodisiac qualities of such things as herbal tea.

Boots is cagey about whether the Nature Boys engaged in any recreational, "natural" drugs, but says that he personally favors just getting "high on life." "I was offered more pot than anyone," Boots says. "People told me, you've got to try it. But my philosophy is, look out for the things that look good, feel good, and taste good. They'll send you up, and send you down."

He is also quick to point out, though, that drug guru Timothy Leary was a fan of his wacky philosophy, and that he doesn't judge folks like Leary. Certainly, the Nature Boys were the predecessors of the hippies and Merry Pranksters of the 1960s as well as the back-to-nature folks of the '70s through today.

According to Boots—as people at Muscle Beach and everywhere else around L.A. would come to call him—there were as many as fifteen Nature Boys living together in the hills around the L.A. area at one time. Boots was particularly close to Gypsy Gene, an accordion-playing bon vivant whom Boots says he met up with by chance while hiking in the hills one day in the 1940s.

Gene was a kindred spirit. Like Boots, he was living outdoors, letting his beard grow, and eating natural foods. He was creative, too. He hoped to immortalize his lifestyle in print: in the 1940s, Gene was working on a book about the Nature Boys' freewheeling life, to be called "Goat Hill" (named for a particular area where they hung out).

Gene gave a peek at the book-in-progress to some of the musclemen at the beach, including Armand Tanny. "I'll tell you, it was going to be a big seller. It was really something," Tanny said of the tale, smiling and shaking his head.

But Gene didn't live to see the book to completion. Boots will say only that Gene was murdered; the story goes that Gene was having an affair with a married woman, whose husband had warned Gene to stay away or else. One day, the jealous husband supposedly caught them together, pulled out a gun, and killed Gene on the spot.

Some say Boots took the name "Gypsy" after Gypsy Gene, as a way of remembering him. Up until Gypsy Gene's untimely death, Boots had been known by a variety of names, including Figaro Boots and even Tarzan Boots. Boots, though, says the name Gypsy Boots was given to him by his friend Don Sargent.

Sargent was another colorful character, known as the "singing sandal-maker" of L.A.'s Fairfax Avenue. He ran a sandal shop by day, where he kept his guitar hanging on the wall; he'd occasionally take it down to serenade customers and passersby. By night, he was a troubadour at small venues around the city. Boots says one day Sargent took out his guitar and made up a song in which he gave Boots the name Gypsy Boots. The name stuck.

The one who would end up spreading the fame of the Nature Boys into mainstream America, though, was a young man called Eden Ahbez. Like Gypsy Gene, the Brooklyn-born Ahbez (pronounced AH-bee) would keep the name he was born with a closely guarded secret throughout his life.

Boots said that after meeting each other in a Los Angeles health-food store, he and Ahbez roamed around together for two years, living between the beach and Tacquitz Canyon near

Palm Springs, with other Nature Boys. They got around in Boots's "Jungle Jeep," an old jalopy that they would sometimes dress up with bunches of bananas and other fruit, hanging where the canvas roof had once been.

Boots became an unofficial leader of sorts of the Nature Boys sheerly because he had the wheels. The Jeep was beat-up but serviceable, making it (although barely, sometimes) as far as San Francisco. (Even back then, the City by the Bay was a home and haven to many unconventional characters.)

Ahbez and Boots shared a love of music. It was Ahbez, a drummer, songwriter, and poet, who would make the biggest name for himself—eventually appearing in national magazines of the time—by penning the Nat King Cole hit single "Nature Boy."

Even in the era of goofy novelty songs, Nat King Cole's 1947 recording of "Nature Boy" stood out as an oddball hit. Lushly orchestrated with strings and a flute solo, the wistful ballad, having few lyrics and lasting less than three minutes, started with Cole crooning about a "very strange, enchanted boy"—sad but wise—who wandered the world.

Somehow, the song struck a chord with listeners in the late 1940s. It had the whimsy of many wartime songs, but also had an exotic quality that was popular in postwar pop music. Perhaps celebrating America's new dominance on the world stage and appealing to men who had gotten the opportunity to see the world for the first time during wartime, popular music at the time was immortalizing such locales as South America and the South Pacific.

Still, the fact that Ahbez got the song to Cole and scored a hit with his first published song was remarkable. He had been living with the Nature Boys and penning songs for several years when he got the courage to try to get some of his creations into the hands of Cole—one of the era's most popular singers.

Cole had recently scored smash hits with "For Sentimental Reasons" and Mel Tormé's instant classic "The Christmas Song." Ahbez figured Cole's hit-making track record and his smooth way with a ballad would make him a natural to sing his songs. Also, Ahbez told *Time* magazine in 1948, "I like the gentleness with which he [Cole] plays."

According to both Boots and the liner notes to *The Nat King Cole Story* on Capitol Records, Ahbez decided to go straight to the source by going to see Cole at a concert date in Los Angeles. According to the Capitol notes, by Leonard Feather:

> Eden Ahbez, who brought this and other songs backstage to Nat at the Lincoln Theater in Los Angeles, would never have gotten to see him had not an intermediary reported some details of Ahbez's unique, almost saintly appearance. A long-bearded figure with flowing robe and sandals, he presented Nat with a variety of unconventional tunes, one of them entitled "I'm a Gone Yogi" and supposedly autobiographical.

Actually, several other accounts say that Ahbez didn't get to see Cole that night; instead, he left the songs with the doorman at the theater. Cole had a look at them and immediately recognized "Nature Boy" as a standout. He then set about tracking down Ahbez and offered him a contract for the song.

"Nature Boy" was said to be part of a suite of six songs about the Nature Boy philosophy and lifestyle that Ahbez had written and presented to Cole. *Time* quoted a lyric from one of the others, titled "Brother Song": "If he's black or white or brown or red or yellow, Just give him love and he's a real good fellow." This one wasn't destined to be another "Nature Boy"—it was, perhaps, both too controversial and too loopy.

Cole never recorded "I'm a Gone Yogi" and the others, but "Nature Boy" turned out to be a big hit, shooting to the top of the charts. It sold nearly a million copies and appears on many Cole "best of" compilations to this day.

Ahbez made tens of thousands of dollars off the song—an estimated $20,000 in the first month alone—and became an overnight media sensation. Within a month of the song's first broadcast on radio, Ahbez was featured in the pages of *Time, Newsweek,* and *Life,* held up as the curious creator behind the quirky song that everyone was listening to.

The skinny, bearded Ahbez was pictured signing autographs for clean-cut teenage fans. Others photos showed him enjoying nature solo and with his pretty wife, Anna Jacobson. He apparently met Anna, who shared his love of nature and natural foods, at the same health-food store where he'd met Boots.

Ahbez's Christ-like visage also adorned big promotional posters for the song. He was the celebrity du jour, even more exotic because he embodied a philosophy that was so out of sync with the straight-laced, conformist postwar society at large.

"Born in Brooklyn," wrote a *Life* magazine reporter, "of parentage as mysterious as his name (both of which he refuses to discuss), Ahbez walked across the U.S. eight times before settling in California's great outdoors with wife, sleeping bag, juice squeezer and bicycle." Wrote a *Newsweek* reporter, "Not too many other men let their hair grow long, go barefoot, meditate, sleep outdoors and eat neither flesh, fish nor fowl."

The press had a field day with Ahbez's bearded and barefoot appearance, his Eastern-influenced philosophy ("As long as I have God in my heart, what need have I for religion?"), and the fact that he didn't use any uppercase letters in his name (he spelled it eden ahbez, saying "only God and the infinite should be capitalized").

After the fad passed, though, he was really never heard from again. Most of his compositions were probably too "out there" for the general public; in any case, none of his other works were turned into hits by a big star like Cole. Ahbez settled into a quiet, comfortable life with his wife and son in the Palm Springs area.

Much later, it was reported that the haunting tune to "Nature Boy" had been lifted from a Hebrew hymn. Ahbez's brother-in-law, A. H. Jacobson, told the press that the matter had been settled out of court, and that the song rights remained with Ahbez.

Ahbez died at the age of eighty-six in 1995, from injuries sustained in a car accident in the desert near Palm Springs. He was said to have still been working on various songs, poems, and a book at the time of his death. Both his wife and son had already passed away before him, so he left no survivors.

Even in 1995, nearly half a century after his one hit song, Ahbez was still well known enough to rate a substantial obituary in the *Los Angeles Times*. Ahbez truly had left a mark on popular culture with that one song and put the Nature Boys in the limelight.

"Nature Boy" helped spotlight the Nature Boys, but it also apparently stirred up some rivalry between himself and his real-life, nature-loving brethren. Even among those who espouse universal love and peace, there apparently is a good amount of professional jealousy. Boots says that after the song became a big hit, Ahbez accused him of trying to steal his thunder.

"Everyone called me Nature Boy. Then he wrote the song," says Boots, who is generally upbeat and energetic almost to the point of being manic. When he discussed Ahbez, though, he seemed genuinely a bit hurt and saddened by their rift. "When Ahbez got real famous, he said I was trying to exploit the song 'Nature Boy.' I said, 'When you were in New York in the basement or wherever playing drums, I was out in nature with long hair, with other Nature Boys.' There was Maximillian [a Yugoslavian immigrant who had a tiny ranch in Calabasas, California, where Boots often hung out]. There was Jesus. Before that, the wrestlers [which Boots pronounces "wrasslers"] were Nature Boys. So nobody owned the name.

"He loved me until he got famous, got in *Life* magazine, and got money," Boots concluded agitatedly. "Money changes people, I suppose."

Still, Boots admitted he admires Ahbez's famous song. "That song has meant a lot to me," Boots wrote in his own autobiography. "What he says is very important and true. *The greatest thing you'll ever learn is just to love and be loved in return* [that is the final line of the song's few lyrics]. Good advice, whether or not you are a nature boy."

For his part, Boots soon became famous, too. His medium was television, as a frequent guest on Steve Allen's pioneering variety show. In some of his dozen or so appearances, Boots would bring his own frenetic health boosterism onstage, blending fruit-and-vegetable concoctions for Allen to sample.

In real life, Boots revealed, Allen was one of a number of Hollywood celebrities who genuinely tried to "follow the way of health." On camera, though, Allen played Boots's appearances for laughs, knowing most people would see Boots as a wacko even if he did make a great fruit smoothie. In 1965, Allen recalled Boots's appearances on his show:

> Since only our comedy sketches and musical numbers were rehearsed—however haphazardly—and the rest of the program was completely extemporaneous, my own as-

tonishment at the way some of our guests comported themselves was not only genuine but shared by the audience, which was ordinarily amused.

Astonishment is certainly the proper word in the case of Gypsy. I shall never forget how on each of his many appearances he came bounding out on the stage with the energy of a dozen men, carrying loads of organic fruits and vegetables and what-have-you, spouting poems with random rhymes and evanescent meter, dancing like Jose Greco on a hot griddle, flying about the stage with carefree disregard of the ability of cameras and microphones to report his activities, and in all throwing our theater into immediate uproar.

Boots was well suited for live TV. He gave the format a needed kick in the pants with his spontaneity, and thrived on the reaction of the audience. His love of the audience was apparently returned: according to Boots, young people in twenty-five cities started Gypsy Boots fan cubs following his appearances on Allen's show, and would demand that he be featured more often when his visits to the show slacked off.

Other times Boots appeared as a musical guest on the show as part of his trio, Gypsy Boots and the Hairy Hoots. The Hoots were two bearded, cowboy-hat-wearing Midwestern boys who met up with Boots in a coffee shop and decided to form a group. They would play guitars while Gypsy sang, played rhythm instruments like the maracas and tambourine, and made a general racket. In addition to guesting on the Allen show, the trio toured the country as part of the *Hollywood Hootenanny* show, and made some other local appearances around L.A.

Even though he led an unconventional lifestyle, Boots did eventually get married in the 1950s. He met his wife, Lois Bloemker, in San Francisco. Her sister introduced the two as a joke on her sibling, and was floored when they hit it off. It must have been quite a shock to see sis fall for a scruffy, wacky man with ill-fitting clothes and no real job. But Boots always did have great energy and magnetism that attracted other people, both male and female.

In fact, there is a quality about Boots—which he surely cultivates—that makes other people want to help him out and take care of him. Boots said that when he, his wife, and young sons later rented an apartment near the beach in Santa Monica, comedian Doodles Weaver—who was actually from a wealthy family, the brother of broadcast honcho Sylvester "Pat" Weaver and uncle of future actress Sigourney Weaver—helped them pay the rent, because he admired Boots's easygoing outlook on life.

The couple would eventually rub shoulders with a number of famous Hollywood folk. Lois was trained as a dancer, and though she wasn't as wild as Boots, she would perform with him at a small health-food stand they opened in Los Angeles. The couple eventually had three sons, all of whom went into the arts (two as musicians, one as a filmmaker).

It was at his Health Hut, located in the West Hollywood area of Los Angeles, where Boots made further Hollywood connections. He recalls such people as Danny Kaye, Gloria Swanson, and Angie Dickinson stopping by to dine on natural foods and juices in an extremely casual setting—apple crates served as chairs.

The souvenir menus described the Health Hut as "a haven for movie moguls, folk singers, fire-walkers, fan dancers, phrenologists, philosophers, psychologists, soothsayers, saints, showmen, space people, professors, poets, phony wrestlers, oppressed quiz show contestants, anthropologists, artists, astrologers, alchemists, yogis, bongo and balalaika virtuosos, tree-dwellers, radical intellectuals, Venusians, and utopians."

Early on, Boots even had a little pet monkey named Peanuts,

who had free run of the place. That ended one day, he claimed, when the monkey swung down from the rafters and landed in a customer's soup. The customer was not amused; neither, surely, was the Board of Health.

But after three years in business, it wasn't the Board of Health that did Boots in, rather it was the typical challenges of running a restaurant. "I gave away more than I sold and the landlord said I was making too much noise," lamented Boots. The Hut was shut.

Boots's celebrity connections have stood him in good stead even after the Hut closed, though. A relentless crusader and promoter, Boots was still showing up into the new millennium at virtually every parade and public event in Los Angeles, beads around his neck and tambourine in hand. He's hobnobbed at various events in recent years with everyone from James Garner to Magic Johnson to (pretrial) O. J. Simpson.

His family doctor, supporter, and friend is Dr. Paul Fleiss—whom Boots knew long before others came to know him as the father of infamous "Hollywood Madam" Heidi Fleiss. According to Boots, Fleiss has high praise for his patient's health. He quotes Fleiss as saying that he has "set new standards of health for senior citizens," and that Fleiss has never known him to be ill "one day in my thirty years of being his personal physician."

Boots is a one-man promotional dynamo for both himself and for Kyolic odorless garlic, a product sold by his cousin Charlie Fox. He's often photographed wearing shirts emblazoned with the Kyolic name. His white van is painted with ads for the firm: "It's ENERGY! It's LIFE!" shout a couple of the statements of praise.

On any square inch of the van that isn't covered by plugs for Kyolic are messages rooting on local sports teams. Boots is often seen creating a stir with his shtick at various sporting events around town. He loves it when the cameras pick him out of the crowd, and local fans call his name. Football is his first love, but in the absence of an L.A.-based NFL franchise, Boots has branched out to baseball, basketball, and hockey games.

He also throws a big birthday party each year: "Not for me, for my friends." Naturally, he invites the local press and TV news crews to cover the events.

On the flyer for his eighty-ninth birthday party, held at Paramount Studios in 1999, Boots gave a "special thanks" to actor Michael Douglas. Michael is the second generation of his family to know the offbeat Nature Boy; Boots met Kirk Douglas when delivering fresh fruits and nuts to his house decades ago, and has since often spent time and played tennis with both generations of Douglases. Wrote Boots to Michael Douglas on his birthday invitation: "Thanks for the cameo in your movie *The Game.*"

Only in L.A. could a ninety-year-old Nature Boy rub shoulders with second-generation Hollywood royalty. Though many at the beach considered him and his friends nutty, Boots has carried on, in his own way, some of the tradition of carefree fun that existed at the original Muscle Beach.

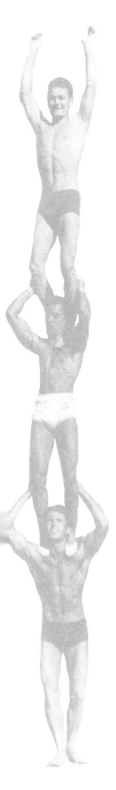

9

Into the Mainstream

Television and World War II were the best things that ever happened to the fitness movement in America. Both brought people together, in a sense, and exposed them to ideas and other people they never otherwise would have encountered. One of those ideas, which had been percolating for some time now, was strength training.

Thousands of men had already gotten into weight training in the 1930s, encouraged by publications such as *Strength & Health*. When these men were called into service in the war, they brought their weights and their passion for training with them. Each enthusiast got at least two or three others, often many more, interested in training to build their bodies and help pass the time.

It was also in the best interests of the military

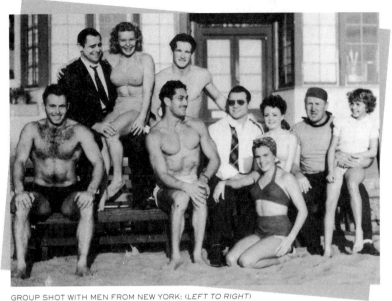

GROUP SHOT WITH MEN FROM NEW YORK: (LEFT TO RIGHT)
DEFOREST "MOE" MOST, STEVE STANKO, PUDGY STOCK-
TON, RUSS SAUNDERS, AN UNIDENTIFIED MAN (SEATED),
JOHN GRIMEK, PEGGY MCFATRIDGE, AN UNIDENTIFIED
WOMAN, JOHNNY COLLINS, BEVERLY JOCHER. (JOE
MAHALIC)

to have the fittest troops possible. The government made training films aimed at both men and women at the start of the war,
stressing the importance of fitness and general health to the war
effort (the series of films also included some that strongly cau-
tioned GIs about venereal disease, and encouraged them to take
advantage of their monthly ration of condoms and the health
services at their disposal). These short films reinforced the idea
that physical fitness was not just desirable, but something one
owed to one's country.

Several of the men associated with Muscle Beach were given
responsibilities in the military that included overseeing physical
training. Fitness and weight training were encouraged on military bases, navy ships, and anywhere else weights could be used
by servicemen.

By the war's end, there were tens of thousands more weight-training enthusiasts than there had been prior to the war. It was natural that the men who came back hooked on training would go on to encourage others to take part: in their jobs, as school-teachers and coaches, and among their own families, they spread the word about fitness and exercise.

Team sports as recreation and character-building activities had long been popular for young men in the United States. What was different now was an emphasis on fitness for its own sake, practiced individually and thought of as a lifelong goal. This was something everyone, from the businessman to the housewife, could do to better their lives, their looks, and their health.

Some of the more progressive-minded men got their wives and girlfriends into working out with weights as well. But many women got hooked on fitness through television. The top cheerleader, salesman, and evangelist for exercise on TV was frequent Muscle Beach visitor Jack LaLanne.

LaLanne hit local TV in 1951. Broadcast from his hometown of San Francisco, he started to get picked up in a number of ma-jor markets around the western United States. In 1959 his show went national, broadcasting from Hollywood to more than two hundred stations across the country. "Stop! Look! Listen! It's time for the Jack LaLanne show, from Hollywood!" exhorted the announcer at the outset of the show, echoing LaLanne's drill-sergeant-like directness and intensity.

Though his wasn't the only fitness show on TV in the 1950s—there was a scattering of local shows—his was the most famous and influential. LaLanne, human dynamo and relentless promoter, rocketed to national fame from his program.

LaLanne would appear in his trademark, skintight dark jump-suit, encouraging viewers to join in with him. He would go through a quick series of exercises, talking to the audience while peppy electronic organ music played in the background.

The program clearly targeted women, with many exercises designed for trimming the thighs and toning the bust. LaLanne would even appeal to kids to get their mothers to exercise with him: he told kids to go get Mom, and tell her "Jack LaLanne has a lot of things to show you, and tell you!"

The show's format, with LaLanne performing exercises while talking to the camera (and never appearing to get short of breath), was a perfect marriage of performer and medium. LaLanne had a gift of gab; he could nearly knock you off your feet with the sheer force and torrent of words coming out of his mouth. "Don't touch that dial!" "Are you with me?" he would periodically chide the audience.

One former Muscle Beach colleague joked, "Someone told me recently they'd had a conversation with Jack LaLanne. I said, 'Oh, really? Because I've known Jack for more than fifty years. And in all that time, I've never had a conversation with him. He talks, and you listen.'"

LaLanne had many followers who wouldn't otherwise have exercised. Many women who wouldn't have felt comfortable joining a gym felt more inclined to give exercise a try at home. Moreover, he presented exercises that used items found in the home as equipment or no equipment at all.

LaLanne's show, though, was even popular among those who did join the growing legions of gym members. "All the women that came to our clubs in the '50s were watching Jack at home," Pudgy Stockton remembers.

The fitness movement couldn't have had a more energetic champion than LaLanne. He didn't just rise to the top naturally—he worked hard at becoming its best-known spokesman. He developed a mythology around himself, spinning a story of his early days that was probably a bit exaggerated. This is how LaLanne tells his story on his Web site:

As a kid, I was a sugarholic. I was a junk-food junkie! It made me weak and it made me mean. It made me sick. I had boils, pimples, and I was nearsighted. Little girls used to beat me up! Mom prayed . . . the church prayed. At the age of fifteen when I heard pioneer nutritionist Paul Bragg speak at the Oakland City Womens' Club in the San Francisco Bay Area, I finally realized that I was addicted to sugar.

Those who know LaLanne say his mother actually knew a thing or two about nutrition herself—it was she who brought Jack to the lecture that day and helped inspire him to take a premedical course in college. But like Charles Atlas and his story about having sand kicked in his face, then returning to face down the lifeguard who did it, this story of LaLanne's seems calculated for conveying maximum humiliation (getting beaten up by girls), followed by a self-created turnaround. It would have been less dramatic to have been the punching bag of little boys rather than little girls, or to give his mother more credit for his eventual success.

LaLanne graduated from chiropractic college, but was "more interested in helping people with precaution, before they became ill." That's when he decided to open his first gym, at the age of twenty-one.

Even without his carefully spun mythology, LaLanne was an unlikely hero. He was on the short side (many bodybuilders and gymnasts were small in stature, generally topping out under five-nine) and had a deep dimple on one knee, apparently the result of an injury he never discussed with his colleagues at Muscle Beach.

To the outside world, LaLanne preferred to appear superhuman and invincible. He couldn't stand to be beaten at anything, always setting out to demonstrate his superiority in any physical challenge. He was a fast-talking, talented, and great-looking athlete, but just one of many standouts at Muscle Beach.

The qualities that really set LaLanne apart were his incredible drive and knack for marketing—what *Sports Illustrated* called in 1981 a sense of "ain't-this-a-kick-in-the-head . . . an ability to communicate a joy in performing" that only a special few in the field of sports and entertainment have. It's a quality that separates popular-but-passing stars from superstars, who will stand the test of time to become icons.

That *Sports Illustrated* article recounted the ways LaLanne promoted himself in the early days:

> By day, LaLanne would parade endlessly in tight T-shirts—"I was in a constant state of flex"—making the scene at all the muscle beaches. He'd leap into a handstand if anyone so much as blinked at him. . . . He was no less visible by night. "I bought the best car I could afford," he says, "plus some really nifty tailored clothes—tight-fitting, to emphasize my chest and shoulders. I dated the very best-looking girls, and I made sure that we were seen at all the best restaurants in town."

LaLanne's formula for getting noticed worked. He still has the knack today. On his Web site, LaLanne manages to call himself "The King of Fitness," "America's Number 1 Physical Fitness Expert and Guru," and "The Godfather of Fitness," all within a couple of paragraphs. On the site, he sells T-shirts, caps, videos, books, and audiotapes of himself and wife Elaine LaLanne.

His "birthday feats" were another example of LaLanne's marketing genius. At the age of forty-one, LaLanne swam the two miles from the island of Alcatraz, home of the famous prison in San Francisco, to Fisherman's Wharf—handcuffed. At sixty,

LaLanne repeated the stunt, this time handcuffed, shackled, and towing a 1,000-pound boat.

LaLanne certainly showed the benefits of exercise through these stunts, but also, of course, promoted himself in the process. The stunts themselves were actually throwbacks to the days of touring strongmen, and to earlier marketing geniuses like Charles Atlas. In 1938, for example, Atlas pulled a railroad observation car, said to weigh 145,000 pounds, for 112 feet.

LaLanne's intensity and determination also made him a favorite on the motivational speaker's circuit. By 1981, when the *Sports Illustrated* article came out, LaLanne was reportedly making $4,000 per appearance as a speaker, appearing at engagements in "a skintight tux." He has continued to be a sought-after speaker at events where a pep talk is in order. Everyone knows Jack and is a little awed by his energy and determination.

LaLanne's fitness empire would eventually extend to all kinds of products. He would put his name on nutritional supplements and at-home exercisers. The most famous of his "brand extensions," though, was the chain of gyms that he licensed his name to. Unlike Vic Tanny's, LaLanne's gyms were not owned and operated by him personally. But they were just as influential at drawing people in and spreading his fame in a tangible way across the country.

LaLanne was just one of the people from Muscle Beach who lent his name to a new breed of gyms, ones that were well-lit and featured fancy equipment and décor. By the 1950s, gyms had become more commonplace, and more inviting. It became a way of competing with other gyms: after all, a gym is basically a big room full of equipment. Along with location, style and ambiance become the decisive factors in members' choices of where to join.

No longer cramped, dingy places stocked only with free weights for the use of wrestlers and boxers, they were often now referred to by the more upscale names of "clubs" or "spas." Weight training for athletes slowly became more accepted by school physical education departments (though it would be another couple of decades before girls and the general student body were widely encouraged to pump iron).

New magazines and physique contests began to spring up, backed by companies that sought to capitalize on America's growing interest in fitness. Once there was money and promotion behind it, weight training became even more well-known and popular.

The '50s also became a kind of golden era for the sport of weight lifting. Bob Hoffman, publisher of *Strength & Health* and the force behind York Barbell, was a chief reason the United States was wildly successful in weight lifting at the 1952 Olympic games in Helsinki.

The U.S. team defeated archenemy Russia handily: Peter George, Tommy Kono, John Davis, and Norbert Schemansky all brought home the gold from Helsinki. These men would go on to visit Muscle Beach, wowing audiences with their lifts.

The victory was particularly sweet in its symbolism, given the Cold War rivalry between the United States and Russia. As is the case every time Americans are especially successful in an Olympic sport—be it gymnastics, swimming, or track and field—interest among the general population boomed. Boys wanted to lift weights, to be like their Olympic idols as much as to build their muscles.

It started to become much more common for young men to have a barbell set at home, to work out with in the basement or the garage. York barbells were even being sold by such mainstream retailers as Macy's department store in the late 1940s. Once you made it into Macy's, you were a product for the masses.

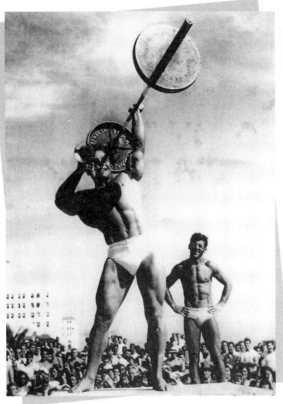

This boom in interest in weight training should have been very good news for Muscle Beach, and in large part, it was. In a way, the popularity of lifting weights was the fulfillment of a wish for many Muscle Beachers, who had worked to spread the positive word of weight training and to dispel myths about it. The beach's fame grew, and there was an even greater emphasis on weight lifting and bodybuilding there.

On the other hand, the dominance of "iron game" sports at Muscle Beach that took hold in 1952–1953 represented the beginning of the end for the original Muscle Beach. At the same time weight lifters and bodybuilders were becoming a main attraction there, the beach's founding acrobats were virtually all leaving. After ten or fifteen years of being regular fixtures there, most felt it was time to move on. They were hitting their thirties, and had the larger concerns of making a living and raising a family. The majority stayed in Southern California, but they moved away from the immediate beach area where they hung out for so long.

The iron gamers replacing them at the beach were a different breed. Gymnastics emphasized all-around athletic prowess and flexibility, and the sport was not controlled by a single, for-profit professional backer. The rise of weight lifting and especially bodybuilding in the United States, backed by Bob Hoffman and Joe Weider, respectively, represented the specialization and professionalization of the sport. By midcentury, many of the men involved in these sports were in it for big stakes, not just for the sheer joy of working out or the hope of getting good enough to become a traveling performer for a while.

As for the iron men themselves, the very thing that made them successful in their pursuits—a solitary, single-minded devotion to winning—made them less social than the acrobats. Furthermore, you can't invite a child up on a platform to play a meaningful part in a bodybuilding exhibition, or to lift hundreds of pounds of weights along with the big boys. And the biggest, heavyweight lifters often appeared . . . how to put this delicately? . . . big and ugly, compared to the lithe acrobats of yesterday.

Those citizens of Santa Monica who had always just tolerated, not supported, the beach area took notice. They didn't understand these newer sports that had become the star attractions of Muscle Beach, and they didn't want to. By the mid-1950s, their sights were set on a way to justify closing the "new" Muscle Beach.

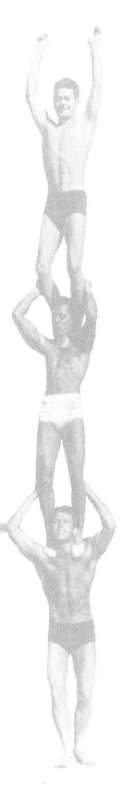

10

The Downfall of
Muscle Beach

The events leading up to the permanent closing of Santa Monica's Muscle Beach have
remained a controversial topic among those who
frequented the beach in its first decade. For the
most part, the alumni of the beach's first fifteen
years still remain either unclear on the reasons—
or willfully ignorant of them.

The old-timers say the beach's closing remains
somewhat of a mystery. Some have theories, others just say they weren't there and don't know
what happened.

Indeed, most of those who were there in the
early days were gone by the late '50s, when the
area was amidst a scandal. Therefore, none of them
probably had firsthand knowledge of the events
that unfolded in late 1958 and into 1959. Also,
the events leading up to the closing were complicated, involving politics, prejudice, and morals

charges. There were many rumors and sensationalized reports in the press at the time.

Some amount of resentment against the famous Muscle Beach had been simmering for years. The biggest gripe of most Santa Monicans was the impossible parking situation created by the weekend throngs. But the more conservative inhabitants of Santa Monica also held a dim view of the presence and growing fame of the beach's muscled, nearly nude men and women. Early on, most had adopted a live-and-let-live attitude.

However, by the mid-1950s, with the mix of people at the beach changing in favor of hulking, heavily muscled weight lifters, the *Saturday Evening Post* ran a splashy, five-page story on Muscle Beach, which was near the apex of its fame. People came from all over the world to see Muscle Beach. Those who couldn't make it personally could send letters addressed simply to "Muscle Beach, U.S.A.," and their missives would arrive at the beach in bulging mailbags.

At that time, there was a hint of trouble brewing between the city and the athletes of Muscle Beach. A few paragraphs into the *Saturday Evening Post* piece, writer Joel Sayre wrote: "Mention Muscle Beach to Southern California's regional cynics, its wise guys, its soft in body, and you are liable to draw only sniggers or snorts."

From the start, there had been some resistance to the installation of the Muscle Beach equipment and platform from the Santa Monica recreation department. A handful of citizens wanted to keep the beach playground for young children only. There was also the resentment of those who resided near the beach, who complained that all the street parking on weekends was being taken up by visitors to Muscle Beach.

These concerns may sound mundane, but they are the stuff that take up countless hours of city council meeting time even in the present day. In fact, these same issues remain hot topics around Southern California today: at some Santa Monica city park playgrounds, there are posted signs requiring that any adult "must be accompanied by a child," in order to discourage vagrants and undesirables from hanging out there. And residents' demand for restricted parking in Los Angeles neighborhoods has boomed—parking in L.A. is a precious and closely guarded commodity.

By the mid-1950s the people of Muscle Beach were a much different group from what they'd been a decade or two before. It wasn't just the faces that changed; more important, it was the bodies and the types of activities. Acrobatics was no longer the rage. Except for a few diehards like Russ Saunders, who still tried to keep the Muscle Beach flame burning despite having a family and a busy career as a movie stuntman, the acrobats had gone on to other pursuits. They weren't replaced by an equal number of newcomers who also performed acts such as hand balancing and adagio.

Instead, fueled by aggressive promoters like Bob Hoffman and Joe Weider, weight lifting and bodybuilding were on the rise. That meant an infusion of pumped-up men—virtually no women or children—who engaged in individual displays and feats of strength, rather than the more communal activities of balancing and tumbling.

By the late 1950s, there were dozens of competing magazines devoted to weight training and bodybuilding. They were of varying quality, and a number had the reputation as being aimed at homosexuals and "perverts." Some who were against the presence of Muscle Beach in Santa Monica no doubt associated everything having to do with bodybuilding with the seamier magazines of the day.

Strength & Health publisher Hoffman accused (probably fairly) his archrival Joe Weider of publishing racy physique magazines aimed at gays. Weider's titles included the colorfully named *Amer-*

ican Manhood, *Body Beautiful*, and *Adonis*. The more hard-core operations, which traded in totally nude photographs and/or ones that were most blatantly suggestive of gay sex or sado-masochism, became targets of ongoing censorship battles with the government.

On the mainstream side, Hoffman saw Muscle Beach as a good promotional tool for his own organization. He sent his lifters there frequently to stage exhibitions. Other lifters went on their own, lured by the Muscle Beach scene.

The large, muscular stature of the bodybuilders and weight lifters was more threatening than that of the earlier Muscle Beach regulars. Many people claimed, as some still do today, to dislike the look of highly developed bodies. The look of skin that has been very deliberately shaved and tanned to a deep glow, stretched over muscles and veins that are much more prominent than the norm, is still shocking to some. The typical cues of what makes one male or female are gone: hairless men with prominent chests and slender waists that somewhat mimic the female form turn traditional standards of beauty on end.

There have been entire books written about the psychology and aesthetics of bodybuilding, including Kenneth Dutton's *The Perfectible Body*. In it, Dutton writes:

> There is a curiously asexual quality discernible in the advanced muscularity of the bodybuilder's physique, and it could be argued that this is a central element in the symbolic language of the developed body. It is not so much that the body is here devoid of sexual connotations, as that it combines in a unique fashion elements of both male and female sexuality.

Of course, most people don't ruminate on the imagery of bodybuilding in such a philosophical manner. To those who derided it, bodybuilding and its attendant conventions—body shaving, posing, the wearing of tiny, tight trunks—simply made men look both too masculine and too feminine all at once. It was "kinky," foreign, creepy.

For many people, it was one thing when a group of sleekly muscled acrobats donned such attire and performed tricks onstage. It was another thing entirely when a lone man stood up and preened for the world to admire him.

In her 1992 book, *The Way We Never Were: American Families and the Nostalgia Trap*, historian/author Stephanie Coontz has an interesting take on what she calls the "sexualization of interpersonal relations." She says that this phenomenon, which began in the 1920s when sexuality "entered the public sphere" and built over the next several decades, accounts for a change in the way Americans viewed anything that could be interpreted as sexual rather than innocent.

"People's interpretation of physical contact became extraordinarily 'privatized and sexualized,'" she writes, "so that all types of touching, kissing and holding were seen as sexual foreplay." Other historians point out that the 1950s saw a rising tide of sentiment against homosexual relations. These two factors combined—the sexualization of physical contact and the campaign against any "abnormal" sexuality—could be seen as contributing to the general discomfort of some people with a place like Muscle Beach in the 1950s.

This was all happening at a time of great, simmering social change—despite our nostalgic image of the innocent 1950s. Girlie magazines like *Playboy* were going mainstream, making the *True Crimes* and *Police Gazettes* of yesteryear look tame by comparison. Women's clothing took on an almost fetishistic shape: tight sweaters, cinched-in waists, form-fitting pants, or exaggerated circular skirts worn over layers of crinolines.

The term *teenager* entered the lexicon as the huge first wave of baby boomers reached adolescence. Adolescence meant rebellion and sex. The older generation fretted even more than previous older generations about youth going to hell in a handbasket. Such songs as "Officer Krupke" from *West Side Story* ("We're a social disease!") and "Kids" from *Bye Bye Birdie* ("I don't know what's wrong with these kids today!") satirized this phenomenon on the Broadway stage.

But it was a serious issue to many adults across America. Santa Monica, staying true to its desire for a small-town atmosphere, tried to keep the devil at bay. The city even banned pinball machines in the mid-1950s, calling them games of chance.

In December 1958, soon after "girlie" magazines started to go mainstream with the appearance of *Playboy*, the Santa Monica city attorney's office and police department cracked down on the sale of "lewd and obscene" photos and periodicals in the city. The mere possession of such material was made a misdemeanor punishable by a maximum fine of $500 and six months in jail. Before 1958, only the selling of "obscene" literature to minors was a crime in Santa Monica. This new strictness was championed by the city's conservative daily newspaper, the Santa Monica *Evening Outlook*. The paper would also turn its sights, on Muscle Beach with a barrage of critical articles and editorials.

The older generation had a great fear and distrust of the youth culture in general, including the growing fascination with muscle for muscle's sake. Sport was fine—nothing wrong, in most fathers' minds by this time, with their boys lifting some weights to train for football or wrestling. But something had to be wrong with these guys who paraded around virtually nude in front of thousands of people. What were they, queers? Perverts?

In 1955, these feelings of distrust, dislike, and anxiety started coming to a head, spurred on by an unfortunate accident at the beach. Even midcentury, the threat of litigation cast a long shadow.

A young boy who wasn't properly supervised picked up a barbell on the Muscle Beach platform. It was much too heavy for him to handle; he fell forward onto it, and hit his head. The boy's parents sued the city, which controlled the Muscle Beach area. The city didn't have insurance for such accidents, and had to cough up an amount equal to thousands of dollars today.

The Santa Monica recreation director told the weight lifters they would have to insure themselves against such occurrences, and do a better job of policing the area—or else the weights would be removed. A Muscle Beach Weightlifters Club was formed, collecting a nominal $2 per year fee from more than 100 members. The money went toward securing Muscle Beach against accidents and lawsuits. This assuaged the city fathers for a time.

But not for long. According to one former Muscle Beach regular, who asked not to be quoted in connection to the events leading up to the closing, old hatreds continued to flare, and be agitated. "There was one kid, 'Hymie' Schwartz [David Schwartz, who in the fifties dubbed himself the "Mayor of Muscle Beach"] . . . who became a loud voice, always agitating the people in City Hall and the recreation department to make improvements to the beach. . . .The head of the recreation department, he didn't like the guys' shape, he didn't like muscle, he didn't like anything. Plus," continued the old-timer, "certain members of the city council were probably just waiting for something to happen down there. As soon as something unfortunately did, they shut it down."

What did happen in late 1958 through 1959 was documented in bold headlines in the *Evening Outlook*. The paper not only sensationalized the events, it quickly rushed to advocate the closure of the beach in the wake of a sex scandal.

According to newspaper reports, five men—two of them top Olympic weight lifters—were charged in December 1958 with sex crimes against children. The charges included contributing to the delinquency of a minor and statutory rape. The actual events were alleged to have occurred in mid-November 1958, in an apartment shared by two of the men near the beach.

Further complicating the issue was the fact that the paper identified the two unnamed girls in the case, said to be twelve and fourteen years of age, as "Negro girls." This was in the days when blacks "had their own beach" further down the coast, as one former Muscle Beach–goer recalled many years later, with obvious skepticism toward the charges. For many people, the race factor was just another facet that made this case particularly ugly.

The two girls reportedly ran away from their Santa Monica home for a week, and ended up spending much of that time in an apartment close to Muscle Beach shared by the weight lifters—who they told police they'd become "acquainted with" before deciding to run away from home. Though headlines termed what happened a "sex orgy," it was a little less dramatic than that—though no less sad, if true. The girls apparently told authorities that they'd been shown obscene pictures and molested by the men.

This was all bad enough on its own. But just five days before the charges against the weight lifters were made public, a Santa Monica jury in an unrelated case awarded a total of $35,000 to four women who had been injured in a landslide on the bluff overlooking the beach several years before. The city was ordered to pay that amount because Palisades Park, the area where the slide occurred and which Santa Monica controlled, was found to be in a "dangerous and defective" condition.

There was immediately talk of closing the park to prevent further such accidents . . . and lawsuits. The park ended up remaining open, following some fairly extensive engineering work. It was a close call, though.

Surely when it came to the case of the runaway girls and the men from Muscle Beach, it must have crossed some bureaucrat's mind that the city might be in big trouble, on top of being caught in a mess of bad publicity, if such a case ever went before a jury. Insurance or no insurance on the part of the Muscle Beach Weightlifters Club, it would never smooth over the taint of alleged sex crimes against children.

Two of the accused "musclemen," as they were described in the paper, were fairly well known. They were Isaac Berger, twenty-two, a world record–holding featherweight weight lifter from the 1956 Olympics, and David J. Sheppard, who took second place in the heavyweight division in the 1956 Olympics. The two had met while training under the auspices of *Strength & Health* publisher Bob Hoffman and his York Barbell company in York, Pennsylvania.

Berger in particular was said to have an eye for the ladies and moved to L.A. partly due to his desire for a freer lifestyle than that imposed by the regimen-loving Hoffman, according to John D. Fair in his book *Muscletown USA*. Fair says Sheppard had been considered one of the most promising young lifters at York, but that he, too, chafed at the restrictions of living at Hoffman's boot camp for champions.

Three other men—John Joe Carper, George Cleveland Sheffield, and William G. Siddall—were also charged in the case. All ended up being exonerated or receiving a slap on the wrist for reduced charges. Berger disappeared for several weeks after the charges came to light. When he eventually resurfaced, he was tried and put on probation for one year. He was also fined $100 for contributing to the delinquency of a minor.

The sentences weren't very stiff, but most of the weight lifters were in fact found guilty of wrongdoing. They ended up dragging down the entire population of Muscle Beach with them.

In the wake of the arrests, Moe Most, a guiding force of Muscle Beach who had been designated a city recreation instructor there, resigned. Though the sentiment wasn't unanimous, some in city government quickly looked to assign blame for the incident to the people of Muscle Beach. The incident was chalked up to a whole culture of alleged perversion there rather than poor judgment or a few "bad apples."

Immediately after the arrests were made in December 1958, there was talk about closing Muscle Beach permanently. "I don't think Muscle Beach is a proper recreational facility," Santa Monica City Councilwoman Alys Drobnick told the *Outlook*. She added, "I've been saying this for the last five years. The Muscle Beach crowd has been bragging about how much publicity they have brought the city. I wonder how they're enjoying the publicity now."

The answer, of course, was that the original Muscle Beach crowd was angry, frustrated, embarrassed, dismayed. Many of them believed the charges were trumped up.

Paula Unger Boelsems and Russ Saunders were among a handful of old Muscle Beach regulars who campaigned to reopen the area. Proposals to the city were made, which promised to address the problems at Muscle Beach while keeping it open.

Most of the old Muscle Beach crowd, though, had moved on with their lives. They either didn't have time to join the crusade to save Muscle Beach or decided not to get involved. Summing up the feelings of most old-timers, Armand Tanny says he didn't join the campaign to save the beach because he saw "the helplessness of it."

Tanny rather bitterly debunks the idea that Muscle Beach was largely attracting a "bad element" by the late 1950s. There were plenty of "groupies," he says, and a few guys who apparently weren't beyond befriending underage girls. But they weren't representative of most people there. Plus, Tanny says, what happened to the area after Muscle Beach was closed was even worse.

"Unfortunately, what happened after they shut down the

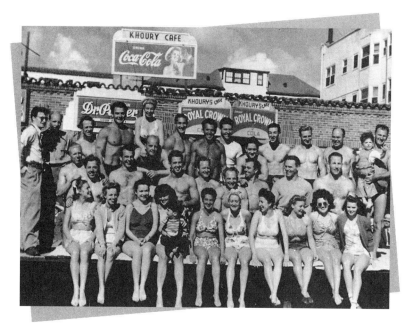

"THE WHOLE GANG," CIRCA 1946. *BOTTOM ROW, FROM LEFT:* HELEN THURSTON, MAXINE CLIFTON, AN UNIDENTIFIED WOMAN, MARIAN ZINKIN WITH HER SON, THREE UNIDENTIFIED WOMEN, PUDGY STOCKTON, IRENE (ROBERTA) MARCYAN, AUDREY SAUNDERS. *MIDDLE ROW:* JUSTUS MOTTER, JOE DE PIETRO (OLYMPIC CHAMPION WEIGHT LIFTER), GLEN JONES, HAROLD ZINKIN, KARRIS KEIRN, GEORGE REDPATH, BRUCE CONNER, WALTER MARCYAN, BOB LEONARD. *TOP ROW:* RAY SAUNDERS, AN UNIDENTIFIED MAN, TIM O'SHEA, GENE AND VERA TESLOF, AN UNIDENTIFIED MAN, DEFOREST MOST, AND THE REST ARE UNIDENTIFIED. THE SMALL BOY AT UPPER RIGHT USED TO PERFORM HANDSTANDS ON THE PLATFORM.

beach was all the dopers from all over Christ's creation came down and made the thing a mess," Tanny says. "The beach became so awful. We would have policed the beach area ourselves."

But a vocal and powerful segment of Santa Monica wasn't interested in giving the athletes of Muscle Beach that chance. One of the more forgiving city councilmen, interestingly, was a minister. The Rev. Fred Judson told the *Outlook* that all the people of Muscle Beach shouldn't be "condemned for the crimes of the few."

Another councilman, Wellman Mills, wasn't quick to rush to

a decision. He said that much of the problem would be addressed through the state's beach acquisition program and the redevelopment plans for the Ocean Park beachfront, which would, in the words of the *Outlook,* "help clean up the area and eliminate the cheap beach apartments inhabited by undesirable Muscle Beach characters."

Still, the *Outlook* played out the scandal for months in large type and overwrought appeals to conservative Santa Monicans to do away with Muscle Beach. It became an all-out crusade for the paper and doubtless helped boost sales. In an editorial that ran the day after Berger was convicted, the paper decried the "beach exhibitionism and riffraff attraction" that Muscle Beach supposedly represented. It snidely remarked on "Muscle Beach athletes and their followers of all three sexes," charging Muscle Beach had become an "attraction for perverts" and "a favorite haven of the sexual athletes and queers of Southern California." The venomous antigay tenor of 1950s America reared its head in the furor over Muscle Beach.

One week later, the paper ran an editorial headlined "You Can Rule Out Muscle Beach." The editorial said they'd collected "hundreds" of ballots from "the majority of the good citizens of Santa Monica," urging the city council not to restore any funds or gymnastic equipment to the beach area. In a strange juxtaposition—given the paper's tirade the week prior about "queers"—the editorial alongside it concerned Liberace prevailing in a libel case against a British paper that implied he was a homosexual. In the case of Liberace, the *Outlook* called the verdict "a reminder to irresponsible writers and publishers that they damage a man's reputation at their peril."

Muscle Beach, as it was, would never reopen.

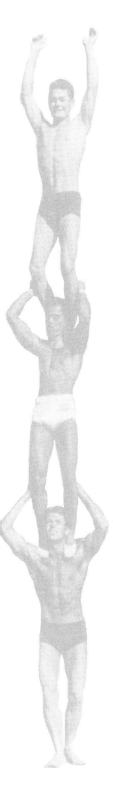

11

The Rise of "The Pit"

Even after the official closing of Muscle Beach, some activity remained near its site on weekends. There was a lawn next to the site where Muscle Beach had been. For years, Russ Saunders, Paula Unger Boelsems, Glenn Sundby, and others would go there, to "the grass" as it was called, to demonstrate and teach acrobatics to others, just as they had on a larger scale during Muscle Beach's heyday. Their affection for gymnastics and commitment to introducing young people to it kept a spark alive.

They would bring basic, portable equipment such as a teeterboard, and put on mini-exhibitions for anyone who would watch. To any who asked, Saunders always remained firm in his assertion that Muscle Beach "never went away."

"We were always here," insisted Saunders in 1998, waving his hand in the direction where the

Muscle Beach platform used to stand. He wore a white shirt, which hung baggily over his thin frame. On the back, he'd silkscreened a photograph of himself in the golden age of Muscle Beach. He was lying on his back, supporting several pretty young women with his arms and legs. "How to Pick Up Girls," read the inscription above the photo. It was a particularly funny sight on an octogenarian.

Saunders was a true believer, who never gave up on the idea of Muscle Beach. He and a few others would continue to champion a return, or at least a recognition, of Muscle Beach the way it once was. They backed a plan, beginning in the late '80s, to encourage Santa Monica to include a "new" Muscle Beach area in its plans to refurbish the beachfront surrounding the pier. That project was finally begun in 1999.

Perhaps Muscle Beach never did leave for Saunders. But to most people, 1959 was the end of the Beach as they knew it, with the removal of the platform and equipment by the city. Bulldozers came in overnight; a parking lot was quickly put in on the eastern edge of what had been Muscle Beach. For thirty years, not even a sign marked the spot where one of Santa Monica's most famous attractions had stood.

After the closing, the weight lifters and bodybuilders had plenty of other places to go. By then, there were many gyms to work out in, so there was no longer as much reason to congregate on the beach. The beach actually made more sense as a gymnastics venue than as a showcase for bodybuilders and weight lifters, anyway.

But those who still wanted to pump and preen under the California sun just packed up their iron and moved a couple of miles south, to the more downscale environs of Venice Beach. Many lifters liked a place to put on a show and work on their tan at the same time. Even before the closing of Muscle Beach, some musclemen had begun to gravitate toward Venice as "their" beach.

By the late '50s, most of the founding members and much of the original spirit that had surrounded Muscle Beach were gone. The popularity of acrobatics had faded, and those who had practiced the sport so well at the beach had left to work and raise families. Also, with the wide embrace of television as a mass entertainment medium, live entertainment in general had begun to occupy a smaller part of people's leisure time. Vaudeville and nightclub work for acrobats dried up.

Meanwhile, weight lifting and bodybuilding had become big business. This was mostly thanks to Bob Hoffman and Joe Weider, two self-styled promoters of the so-called "iron game" sports. The two first started competing with each other for muscles and dollars by the late 1940s, and remained bitter rivals for decades.

Hoffman ran a military-like training center for national-caliber weight lifters in York, Pennsylvania. At his York Barbell headquarters, nicknamed Muscletown, USA, Hoffman gave young men the training they needed to become world champions, along with jobs to help earn some money while chasing their dreams. Hoffman capitalized on and fed his passion for weight lifting by branching out beyond making barbells into products such as high-protein dietary supplements.

Even during Muscle Beach's heyday, Hoffman was sending men around the country, stopping at Muscle Beach and many lesser-known locations, to put on weight-lifting exhibitions and generally spread the word about the sport. There are photographs from the postwar years at Muscle Beach, showing York men like Steve Stanko and John Grimek hanging out with the Muscle Beach crowd. York would also stage publicity stunts, such as giving some of the Muscle Beach strongwomen York shirts to wear while they hoisted York barbells on a platform for the crowd.

By the late 1960s, America's weight-lifting prowess faded—the sport became dominated by Eastern Bloc countries, which threw the resources of the state behind creating Olympic champions. That was bad for Hoffman, who'd staked his empire on the sport.

But as bodybuilding became more popular, Weider pulled ahead to become the dominant force. He founded such contests as Mr. Olympia and created an empire around his shows, publications, and fitness-related products. Unlike weight lifting, bodybuilding was not an Olympic sport—though, over the years, Weider has tried doggedly to get the sport admitted into the Olympics.

But because bodybuilding wasn't an Olympic sport, there were fewer restrictions on what Weider could do businesswise. Also younger than Hoffman, Weider became known as the more aggressive and innovative of the two by the late 1950s. Some columnists and athletes who'd worked for Hoffman switched over to Weider, who offered them sweeter deals.

By the early '70s, Weider would move his operation to California, which he recognized as the present and future capital of bodybuilding. Armand Tanny says he helped convince Weider to set up shop in the west San Fernando Valley town of Woodland Hills, where the company remains based today. It's less than a half hour's drive from there to Malibu Beach.

When weight lifters started congregating in Venice, the sport was still near the height of its popularity. Like Muscle Beach, the Venice weight-lifting area was controlled by the city. But unlike Santa Monica, Venice was part of Los Angeles—a fairly down-at-the-heels part of Los Angeles.

The musclemen apparently had little problem convincing the city to let them set up shop in a small area there called "The Pit" or "The Pen." As the name suggests, the area was little more than an enclosed pen, with barbells and dumbbells inside on a low (not raised, like Muscle Beach's) platform. It wasn't much to look at, but it still had a novelty factor for tourists and Angelenos who came across it at the beach.

Beachgoers started to hang out there, watching the men build their muscles. But except for summer holiday weekends, when The Pen started hosting physique competitions in the manner of the old Muscle Beach, it was more like visiting the zoo than visiting the circus, as going to the original had been. It was more a curiosity than entertainment.

With the arrival of the musclemen, muscle-related businesses soon followed into Venice. Real estate around the beach area remained relatively cheap. Muscle Beach veteran Joe Gold founded Gold's Gym nearby, on Venice's Pacific Avenue, in 1964. The gym established itself as "the Mecca of bodybuilding," as its slogan says, by its association with bodybuilding superstars. Arnold Schwarzenegger worked out there in the movie *Pumping Iron*.

Gold was a native of the heavily Russian East Los Angeles neighborhood that also spawned such Muscle Beach regulars as John Kornoff and Johnny Collins (née Kulikoff). He had spent as many hours as he could at Muscle Beach during his wartime stint in the merchant marine. After the war, he returned to Los Angeles and became a well-known muscleman. He appeared with Armand Tanny, George Eiferman, and the others in Mae West's touring stage show in the '50s.

Gold's Gym became the gym of choice for bodybuilders. Many would use Gold's for their primary workout, and also pay the nominal fee to belong to The Pen, where they could enjoy the scenery and soak up the sun. The two were just a few blocks from each other in Venice.

Arnold Schwarzenegger's arrival in the United States heralded a major turning point for bodybuilding—and helped put Gold's Gym on the map in a much broader way. By the late '60s, bodybuilding was gaining in popularity, but still remained basically a "back of the closet" sport, said Gold.

That's when Weider was introduced to the young Austrian bodybuilder, who'd been having some success in Europe. Weider, seeing Schwarzenegger's potential to become a star and make a lot of money for everyone involved, helped him come to the United States.

Schwarzenegger started building his American dream on the sand in Venice. Lou Ferrigno, later the star of TV's *The Incredible Hulk,* also began making a name for himself at The Pit. The presence of these types of stars, along with *Pumping Iron,* inspired hundreds more aspiring stars to come to Venice. The place gained prestige as a kind of dream factory for bodybuilders, and by the early 1970s, many people were referring to The Pen as Muscle Beach. The annual physique show there was actually called the Muscle Beach Contest.

It had been more than a decade since the original closed. Still, the co-opting of the name ruffled some feathers among Muscle Beach old-timers. A few, like Saunders and Boelsems, had tried for years to get Santa Monica to reinstate Muscle Beach, or at least to give it some recognition. They knew that their Muscle Beach, the original, was in danger of being forgotten; calling another place Muscle Beach was just another step in that direction.

Eventually, those at The Pen wanted to legitimize their status by gaining official recognition of the use of the name Muscle Beach. Making the name official took some time—like the events surrounding the establishment and demise of the original Muscle Beach, proving once again that anything involving politics and city government is a long and tedious process.

In the mid-'80s, Joe Mack was the new "Mayor of Muscle

Beach." It was his job to oversee and promote The Pen as both a well-known recreational facility and the successor to Santa Monica's Muscle Beach.

By that time, the muscle gyms of Venice were not only world-famous, they'd turned into international businesses. They licensed their names and logos around the world, spreading the fame of their gyms and lining their coffers in the process. Gold's Gym had its bald-headed, hulking weight lifter hoisting a barbell sagging under the heavy weights stacked on each end. World Gym, opened by Joe Gold six years after he sold Gold's Gym, had as its logo a big gorilla lifting a barbell.

It was all part of the culture of celebrating the hard-core bodybuilding lifestyle. The fad came with the popularity of Schwarzenegger and TV shows like *American Gladiator*. Even people who had never broken a sweat in a muscle gym started sporting these gyms' licensed goods. They supplied cachet and attitude by association.

Mack saw all of this and decided that Venice's Pen should not only be designated Muscle Beach, it should have its own mascot. He drew up plans to rename The Pen "Muscle Beach Venice," along with a drawing of a nasty-looking, long-fanged boar. The proposed logo was "Muscle Beach Venice: Home of the Hog," with the drawing of a snarling pig's head in the middle. He presented the plan, hog face and all, to the city.

The proposal went over like a lead balloon; the city quickly rejected the idea. The hog logo, they said, might be offensive to some. Plus, there was the possible political issue of people from the original Muscle Beach becoming upset at the use of the name. The city said they couldn't put their stamp of approval on a plan that just co-opted the name.

It was back to the drawing board for Mack. Steve Ford, a young bodybuilder from L.A. who was a freshly minted college graduate with a degree in communications, says he approached

Mack and offered to help. He suggested that they just go for the name Muscle Beach, rather than pushing for the acceptance of the pig logo.

After doing some research and getting through several layers of bureaucracy, Ford was told that in order to approve the name Muscle Beach Venice, the city would need a letter from one of the notable people from the original Muscle Beach, stating that the use of the name was okay by them. Ford was determined to find one, though he wasn't sure at first where to look.

As luck would have it, Ford and Muscle Beach legend Armand Tanny both belonged to a gym in Chatsworth, a community in L.A.'s San Fernando Valley. Ford contacted Tanny through the gym. After hearing Ford's pitch, Tanny, then an editor at Weider's *Muscle and Fitness*, agreed to write a letter on the magazine's letterhead supporting the proposed Muscle Beach Venice name to the city recreation and parks department.

That seemed to do the trick. In May 1987, the city officially renamed The Pen "Muscle Beach Venice." Several years later, the place would get a complete overhaul to help it live up to its reputation. After the *Pumping Iron* glory days, the facility fell into steady decline. In 1991, Muscle Beach Venice reopened a totally new weight-training area, anchored by a barbell-shaped concrete building.

Muscle Beach Venice could never replace or replicate Santa Monica's Muscle Beach, but it has served as a reminder of the original beach's significance in the world of fitness and sport. The drive to get The Pen dedicated as Muscle Beach also reunited many of the old Muscle Beach crowd. They caught up with each other, shared memories, and made another run at getting their Muscle Beach the recognition it deserved.

Many had not seen or heard from each other in the several decades that had passed since their beach days. Many were grandparents by the late 1980s; with their family-raising and working days pretty much behind them, a number of them took up the cause again.

Ford offered to work as a volunteer publicist for the "alumni" of Muscle Beach 1934–1959, after securing their approval for the name change and seeing that project in Venice through completion. In 1987, Glenn Sundby, Paula Unger Boelsems, Harold Zinkin, and Jack LaLanne founded the Muscle Beach Alumni Association. The organization produced newsletters for fellow members, gathered personal histories and photographs from the era, and championed the official commemoration of Muscle Beach by the city.

In 1988, the group submitted a proposal to the city of Santa Monica for a new platform at the original Muscle Beach site. It took a dozen years, but the plans, in a modified form, finally became a reality. There's no actual platform, but there will be a broad lawn on which gymnastics demonstrations can be staged in a better venue than the beach has seen in decades. New rings, parallel bars, and high bars have also been installed at the site, though it's a far cry from the old days, when the place was a bustling and exciting hub of activity.

In 1989 this group of alumni also succeeded in getting the small plaque erected at the site of the original Muscle Beach. Again, it was a bit of a compromise; originally, they had envisioned a memorial that would contain the names of those who were active in the "golden years" of Muscle Beach. But at least the small plaque recognized the site where for years one of the more remarkable and famous places in the history of the American fitness movement had once stood. After all those years and all their individual accomplishments, the alumni of Muscle Beach still wanted to feel legitimized by a physical reminder of Muscle Beach.

With the new area dedicated to Muscle Beach in Santa Monica reopened, the plan is to keep that place dedicated to gymnastics, while Venice will represent the iron sports. Even when Muscle Beach began, there was little distinction between gymnasts and those who worked out with weights—many did both—but the competitive and economic incentives of the sports today have caused them to specialize.

By the time The Pen became known as Muscle Beach, bigger was definitely better, and the bigger guys were the ones who became stars. In pursuit of that, steroids became commonplace, allowing bodybuilders to obtain cartoonishly large proportions. Though the drugs obviously have a downside, the resulting physiques probably helped fuel the huge surge in the popularity of bodybuilding, which continues to this day.

In fact, steroids first started being used by American weight lifters in 1960—one year after the permanent closure of Muscle Beach. The closing, then, marked the end of an era in more ways than one. The introduction of steroids into the iron sports marked the beginning of an entirely different era, one where lifters and bodybuilders began to feel they had to be on "the juice" to be competitive. Men got huge, records were shattered, but who knew how much of this was the result of drugs?

Ironically, a movement that started by preaching the joys of working hard and living clean changed into a culture that was all about how one looked. Bigger at any cost became the dominant way of thinking; the public's fascination with that look spurred hundreds of thousands of "wannabes" to join franchised muscle gyms—or to at least buy the T-shirt.

It also meant that women were either relegated to the sidelines, since they are not as big as men, or were expected to make themselves look like men in order to compete. Steroids can effect particularly dramatic changes to the female physique, creating bodies so heavily muscular and low in body fat that they truly don't look female anymore.

At the other extreme, women became bimbo cheerleaders

for the hugely muscled men. Turn on "professional" wrestling today, and you'll see women who look like refugees from a silicone-enhanced production of "Li'l Abner" playing the wrestlers' molls.

Where did the strong, feminine women of the 1940s go? Hopefully, their likes are starting to reappear in other sports, such as women's soccer and basketball. Meanwhile, the iron sports have unfortunately reverted to being perceived as a men-only domain, even as more and more women from all walks of life take up some form of weight training for fitness.

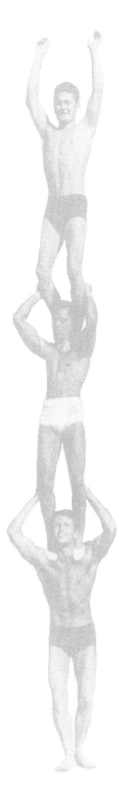

12

Lifelong Fitness

P*sst* . . . want to know the secret to fitness? Combine regular exercise with a diet of fresh, healthful foods eaten in moderation. Repeat this prescription for the rest of your life. That's all there is to it.

That's all the beautiful, fit, healthy people pictured in this book were doing decades ago. They didn't have the benefit of our latest exercise equipment, trendy classes, fashionable supplements, pills, and potions.

The evidence is overwhelming: Americans are fat. A study printed in the *Journal of the American Medical Association* (*JAMA*) in late 1999 stated that more than 40 million Americans, 22 percent of the population, were obese . . . that is, more than thirty pounds over their ideal weight. The pace of weight gain across the country was found to be accelerating at an alarming rate; in a cruel irony, the state of California was found to have the seventh-highest percent increase in obesity from 1991 to 1998. By 1998, the Golden State, birthplace of the American fitness movement, had 66.7 percent more obese people than seven years previous. The consequences are also clear: roughly 300,000 people, according to *JAMA*, die each year as a direct result of obesity. And finally, people are getting fat at younger and younger ages: compare the kids at the local junior high and high school today to the same student bodies of two or three decades ago. There's a lot more heft on campus these days.

Many books, drugstore products, and mail-order products promise miracles. But the biggest secret about the key to fitness is that there is no secret. It may seem old hat, it may not sell as many books and magazines as the latest fad, but the simple truth is that diet and exercise are the only way to achieve good health. It doesn't come in a pill or a bottle. You don't have to spend $30 on the latest, bestselling diet book to discover this.

A lot of people today fail at combining diet and exercise in a regular routine. People will eat processed, low-fat foods but only get to the gym a couple of times a month, then wonder why they're not losing weight. (Answer: because you have to burn off more calories than you take in, and even "low-fat" foods can be fairly high in calories and sugar.) Other folks exercise two or three times a week, but fail to watch what they eat. You can't achieve maximum results either way.

Nutrition seems to be the hardest component for many people. We are conditioned to eat often, individually and in groups, even if we're not hungry. It's not like we don't know that we shouldn't: nutritionists say that most people know what they should do even before consulting them—they just can't seem to do it on their own.

There is no lack of information today on the benefits of fresh, natural food. Unlike sixty years ago, when the Muscle

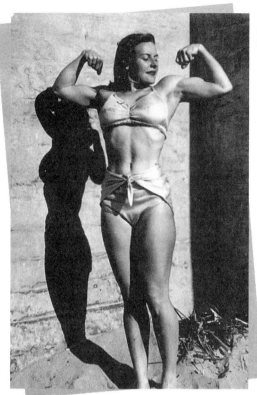

Beach crowd was learning from each other, there are dozens of
mainstream publications, videos, and other sources that are full
of good, useful tips on diet. Yet more than 80 percent of us
don't eat enough fruits and vegetables, and five out of the six
leading causes of death in the United States are related to diet.
Many of us hear these kinds of statistics over and over. We may
try to change our habits for a week, but then lapse back into the
bad habits of our hectic lives, which means subsisting on fatty
snacks and fast food.

Does anyone really need to be told that cheeseburgers and
french fries aren't health food? Information on diet and nutrition is widely available at libraries and doctors' offices today.
We've known the basics for decades, yet people keep searching

for the "silver bullet" that will make diet and exercise easy and pleasant. "Our mouth is our biggest enemy," says George Eiferman, echoing the sentiments of just about everyone else who came out of Muscle Beach.

Theories may come and go about food combinations and the best work-out program, but one can't go wrong with fresh, natural foods and regular, moderate exercise of any type. Walking, biking, swimming, it doesn't matter: getting moving is what counts.

Life extension is a hot topic: everyone seems to be trying to figure out how to stave off death. But doctors will generally tell you that the most desirable goal, and the one you have more control over, is to remain healthy and active until the end of your life—whether that comes at age sixty-five or age one hundred five.

By that measure, the majority of Muscle Beach veterans seem a success. Surely, genetics always plays a role: longevity tends to run in families. On the other hand, there are several instances among Muscle Beach old-timers where the one or two siblings who were active at the beach have far outlived their siblings who were more sedentary.

Active and vital well into their seventies and eighties, the alumni of Muscle Beach aren't the type of people who sit at home, waiting for a letter to arrive or for the phone to ring. They take charge, enjoying such vital pursuits as camping and mountain climbing into ripe old age.

What are their lives like now? They don't look like thirty-year-olds; most have put on a little weight and move more slowly than they used to. But they know what to do, and, to borrow a phrase from a popular athletic-shoe maker, they just do it. Many of the traits we associate with getting older—such as becoming stiff and having digestive problems—can be significantly lessened through proper diet and exercise.

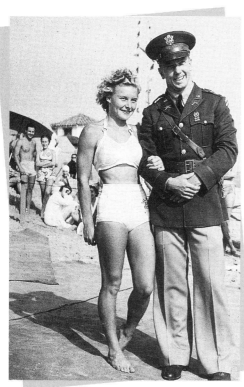

Muscle Beach veterans tend to stay busy both physically and mentally. Les and Pudgy Stockton read a lot and stay on top of current events, in addition to staying physically active. They still live in Santa Monica, just a mile or so from the site of Muscle Beach, in a rent-controlled apartment jammed full of memories. Pudgy keeps scrapbooks of their Muscle Beach and gym-owning days, and plaques and trophies share wall space with family photos.

Les in particular, who's always been known for his sense of humor, is sharp and down-to-earth enough to joke about the people his age who either dwell on death or deny that it exists. He and Pudgy get the most out of the life they've been given, while being realistic about their limitations.

Les enjoys friendly discussion and argument, giving the salesmen and missionaries who often target older people an earful and a well-considered debate if they call on him. Among his many projects, Les Stockton is working on a book about his and Pudgy's adventures in mountain climbing. The couple also collects butterflies, and gives talks about butterflies and insects to school groups. They find great pleasure in introducing kids to the beauty of creatures many just think of as "icky."

The couple still walk and use light weights to stay in shape. When their knees aren't bothering them, they climb Santa Monica's well-known Sixth Street steps, a huge flight of steps that run straight down a canyon hillside. A quick tip: take care of your knees. They are the body part that seems to give these otherwise fit people the most trouble. Many of the people who were at Muscle Beach had knee problems at the time, or developed them later.

Armand Tanny lives in the San Fernando Valley, not far from the offices of his longtime employer, Weider Publications. His daughter's gym, Tanny's Personal Fitness, is also in the neighborhood, part of the suburbs of Los Angeles.

Tanny likes to take trips to the Sierras in his camper. His knee, injured while wrestling, has bothered him most of his life. Still, he's managed to become a champion athlete who's still very active, as well as a renowned writer on fitness. He has continued to work out regularly, and holds memberships to a number of different gyms.

When it comes to exercise, "You don't need a hell of a lot of exercise to be in good shape," Tanny says. "A good twenty-minute workout each day can do more for you than an hour a day, if you're watching your diet," he says, scoffing at the notion some hold today that one has to work out an hour or two per day to be really fit.

Tanny and others agree that diet is the forgotten element for many people who lead otherwise healthy lives today. They join gyms, they don't smoke, but they're not careful about what they eat. It needn't be hard to find the "good" foods; Tanny has a novel take on where to find healthy food in a supermarket. Tanny points out astutely: "All the good foods are around the periphery of the supermarket. You go down the center aisle, and you only see cans and boxes. I don't even go down those center aisles. The good foods are the fresh fruits, fish, and meats."

Ask Tanny why we're getting fatter as a nation, even now that everyone is aware of the benefits of a good diet and exercise, and Tanny goes off on a passionate tangent. "We're a nation addicted to sugar," Tanny says. "It's not fat in our foods that makes us fat—you need fat to process the vitamins . . . but sugar promotes insulin swings, so you can't process food. It causes all kinds of health problems."

Tanny says he sums up his best diet advice for me in two words: "raw food."

Ironically, raw food is a bit of a fad in fashionable cities these days. Organica in San Francisco and SunFire in New York are two of the well-known eateries pushing uncooked fare; Organica's chef, the one-named Juliano, has written a popular "uncook book" full of raw recipes. Muscle Beach alumni like Armand Tanny, George Redpath, and Gypsy Boots beat Juliano to the punch half a century ago.

George Eiferman concurs on the benefit of healthy food. "For the average American, if food tastes good, that's enough for them," he says. "Our greatest enemy is our mouth."

When interviewed in late 1999, Eiferman was in good health, considering he nearly died several years earlier. While living between Hawaii, where he had a gym, and the mainland, he fell gravely ill and was in a coma for weeks. He was divorced at the time, but his ex-wife Bonita Gail stepped forward to care for him and help nurse him back to health.

By 1999, he was back to working out, living again in Las Vegas. In addition to Bonita, he's close to his daughter, who works in a Vegas beauty salon. The lifelong prankster and teacher speaks a little slowly these days, but he knows he's lucky to be alive and to have had the life he's led.

Like Tanny, Eiferman stresses that consistency and moderation can be more valuable than going full throttle. "People try to do too much, too soon," Eiferman says. "Those that last the longest, like Armand Tanny, pace themselves well."

Gypsy Boots has made a career out of playing the nutty clown, but he must be doing something right. He's as fit a ninety-year-old as you'll ever see. "Nuts and fruits for Gypsy Boots," one of Boots's many quips, sums up his diet philosophy.

Boots says he starts the day with exercise and eats healthy food in moderation. "Many people roll out of bed, after lying down all night long, and they go straight from the bed to the table. They're out of their minds," Boots says in his book *The Gypsy in Me!*

Instead, Boots says, "I go out and do some exercise, whether it's jogging, squats, sit-ups, and pushups, walking fifteen minutes, jumping up and down, lying on my back and raising my legs up and down, doing some deep breathing, standing on my head, going to the local gym, or lifting a rock. Just get the blood circulating. Otherwise," he adds, with characteristic puckishness, "you're going to be out of circulation."

Finally, understand that genetics and just plain luck do play a factor. This doesn't excuse being out of shape: many people who could greatly improve their health through exercise and diet fall back on the argument that they're "genetically predis-

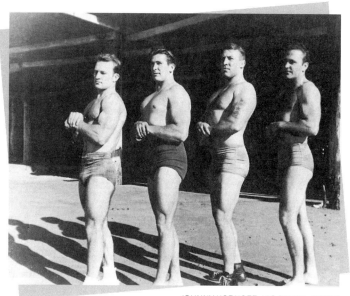

JOHNNY KORNOFF, VIC TANNY, FRANK
JARES, AND GORDON MCRAE POSE
BESIDE THE PIER. (TED O'BRIEN)

posed" to fatness (and by the way, fat is fat—no matter where it is on your body, what it looks like, or whether you call it a "spare tire" or "cellulite"). There may be some rare cases where certain individuals don't respond well to normal weight-control techniques. But for the vast majority of us, they can work. That doesn't mean it is easy.

But at a certain point, if you exercise regularly and eat right, you shouldn't beat yourself up if your health isn't quite as good as Gypsy Boots's at the age of ninety. Longevity is significantly controlled by genetics—which is why the people in some families just seem to live a long time, regardless of whether they smoke or drink or whatever. Again, though, that doesn't mean the reverse is true: that you can smoke a pack a day, and have as good a chance of living a long, healthy life as anyone. The research in that area is pretty clear by now.

As for looking like Steve Reeves or Pudgy Stockton in their

heyday—you also shouldn't expect miracles here. Even fellow athletes, who worked out just as hard alongside these remarkable specimens, describe the natural endowments of these beautiful bodies as "one in a trillion." Many of the entertainers, particularly women, we see in the media today fall back on surgery to create fuller bosoms, flatter tummies, and sleeker thighs. Very few are born to perfection.

The explosion of cosmetic surgery doesn't simply reflect a desire to get more beautiful the "easy" way: it also is an admission that there are certain limitations to what most of us can achieve through training. The popular look today of women with large, round breasts and sleek, even scrawny, hips and legs is actually an unnatural, unattainable goal for the majority of females.

Honest people who make their living as personal fitness trainers will tell you that they can work out all day, every day and still not have the ideal body that they'd like. Exercise isn't going to make you grow a chest like Stockton's, or have the same bone structure as Reeves. Men with long, lanky builds aren't going to look the same as shorter men with stocky builds will as they develop their bodies.

But . . . here's the good part . . . virtually anyone can improve their looks AND their health through exercise and weight training. That was the revelation that drove the people of Muscle Beach to spread the word, and prompted millions of people to follow their example. Skinny kids grew up to be Mr. America. Sickly kids became professional acrobats. Most important, they gave themselves full, healthy lives through exercise.

Quite simply, it works. It's not easy, but it's simple. And it doesn't have to cost much, except in terms of determination and commitment.

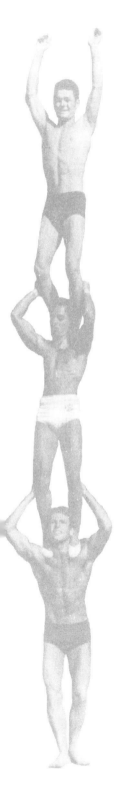

EPILOGUE

Present and Future

Though its demise was unfortunate, Muscle Beach was only the beginning. Today, tens of millions of people, both men and women, belong to gyms. Many millions more take part in sports and exercise on their own: walking, biking, running.

In the heyday of Muscle Beach, seeing someone running down the street in sneakers and sweatclothes would have been reason to call the cops—or at least look askance at the person as a "health nut." Today, even people who rarely lift a finger like to brag about their "workouts."

Vic Tanny showed that opening a nationwide chain of dozens, even hundreds, of gyms was possible. Again, it is unfortunate that his empire crumbled and left some customers with long-term memberships and nowhere to go. But Tanny paved the way for convenient, pleasant, affordable gym chains everywhere. For the average person, comfort and variety make a tremendous difference in motivating them and keeping them interested in working out, so this was an important advance.

People like Harold Zinkin and Walter Marcyan marketed the machines that would fill these gyms. As with gym ownership, there were other people doing it. There may even have been other machines over the years that came first, or were more advanced. Again, though, the contribution of these Muscle Beach alumni was important because they were successful at it, and marked a path for others. The availability of prefab gym machines, in turn, made it more feasible to open more gyms around the United States.

The women of Muscle Beach helped to promote exercise and fitness for other women. They showed you can be strong, athletic, competitive, and still beautiful and feminine. We've long celebrated famous women of sport, including such stars as Sonja Henie and Babe Didrikson, but for years they were treated as an aberration: a once-every-four-years sideshow at the Olympics.

Today, after years of both advances and setbacks, we are finally starting to see this ideal become a viable, ongoing reality. Little doll-sized girls who skate and tumble at the Olympics are still among the biggest stars, but big, strong women who compete in soccer, basketball, and weight lifting are also moving into the mainstream as role models. They offer girls a whole new set of ideals to aspire to.

Weight lifting in particular, long considered purely a male sport by most of the public, is opening up for women. Women's weight lifting was an Olympic competition sport for the first time ever in the 2000 Olympics in Sydney, Australia. Getting a sport into the Olympics is the goal of all sports boosters, because it gives such instant visibility and credibility to the sport.

Just as Pudgy Stockton's pretty face and fantastic figure made her a poster girl for women's fitness and weight training mid-century, women's weight-lifting boosters have hoped an attractive young woman would give that sport some sex appeal. In an interview with *USA Today* two years before the games, weight-lifting coach John Thrush admitted, "We have an image problem . . . our sport in general is misunderstood. It's tenfold bad with women. It's been such a hard sell. Let's face it. Image and the way people look—we're talking charisma—is incredibly important. If they see someone . . . who is fit, but not a monstrous person, she can change a lot of stereotypes."

Thrush coached Melanie Kosoff-Roach, a comely and petite former gymnast from Sumner, Washington, whom *USA Today* called a "5-foot, 126-pounder with a face you could find in the pages of *Vogue.*" Though Kosoff-Roach garnered a lot of press and was considered a strong contender for the Olympic team, she failed to go to Sydney in 2000—unfortunately for her, Thrush, and perhaps the image of the sport among Americans.

The United States did have a particularly strong contender in Savannah, Georgia, native Cheryl Haworth, however. Haworth was among the top finishers among the female heavyweights. In the midst of coverage dominated by small and cute female gymnasts, soccer players, and runners, though, Haworth and her teammates were not able to make much of a ripple in U.S. national Olympics media coverage. Still, the very fact that they were there was a positive step for women's sports.

Bodybuilding, meanwhile, became so popular by the 1980s that its aesthetic pervaded entertainment. There was Schwarzenegger (of course), *American Gladiators* on TV, and a huge resurgence in wrestling—this time around, with wrestlers who were obviously pumped up through bodybuilding. Bodybuilders also became popular with ad agencies, to hawk everything from food to household appliances.

The big difference with bodybuilding today is steroids. These muscle-building drugs have legitimate medical applications; in fact, they were developed in the 1930s for use in treating the weak and elderly. Today, steroids are often found in such things as prescription allergy medications. But once bodybuilders saw what steroids could do for their bodies, muscle enhancement became the drugs' best-known application.

The "steroid era" began in 1960, when several weight lifters began taking Dianabol, an anabolic steroid, under the supervision of Dr. John Ziegler. Ziegler worked with lifters at York and other clubs on various training methods. Few things had ever improved strength and size so quickly as the steroids did. When others witnessed the success of these athletes, they followed suit.

The use of steroids by weight lifters and bodybuilders became common by the late 1960s. It wasn't until the 1976 Olympics that athletes were tested for the drugs; more weight lifters tested positive than any other types of athletes. In following years, though, athletes in other sports have been revealed to be "on the juice," from track stars to cyclists.

Most people are aware that steroids are widely used among football players and wrestlers today. The almost universal use of steroids in professional bodybuilding today is one major reason why there's little hope of the sport as it exists being admitted into the Olympics. If subjected to Olympic-style drug testing, virtually all competitive bodybuilders would be disqualified. There are "natural" bodybuilding competitions, but these don't get nearly the financial support or the notice that the mainstream contests do.

It's not just professional and competitive athletes with their whole careers on the line who are turning to steroid use. Today, young people, mostly males, in college and even high school start taking the drugs to gain an edge. Many argue that, with everyone on steroids, you have to join them or be left behind.

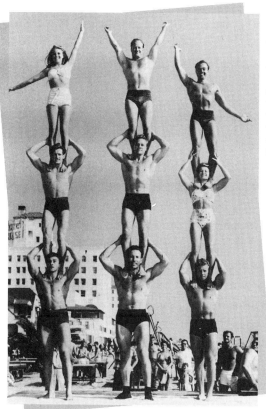

THREE THREE-HIGH
TOWERS: LEFT TOWER:
BOTTOM, ALEX JACKSON;
CENTER, RUSS SAUN-
DERS; TOP, UNIDENTIFIED
GIRL. RIGHT TOWER: BOT-
TOM, LES STOCKTON; CEN-
TER, PUDGY STOCKTON;
TOP, BRUCE CONNER.
(CENTER TOWER: THREE
UNIDENTIFIED MEN.)

Some Muscle Beach alumni shrug, and say they would have used steroids if they'd been available. Clearly, they work if your goal is quick muscle gain. But others are set against the drugs, pointing to possible adverse health effects and the simple notion that one should compete on an even playing field. It does take the joy out of sports for many of us when we're left to speculate how much of an athlete's accomplishments are "natural" and how much are attributable to drugs.

Historian and writer Jan Todd summed up the feelings of the antisteroid camp in a 1990 editorial in *Iron Game History*: "Even though anabolic steroids produce results, they do so at the cost, in the case of bodybuilding, of the very thing which has always been the bedrock of bodybuilding—a healthy lifestyle. How ironic it is for a man to take steroids so that he can stand on a posing platform as a symbol of health. One of the things about bodybuilders in the presteroid era that stood out . . . was their vibrant good health."

Ultimately, we can't know the full effect that everyone from Muscle Beach has had, as they've gone on to found gyms, market equipment, or teach others. Who can say how many kids started working out, became athletes, or merely developed more of an appreciation for sport and the capabilities of the human body after hearing George Eiferman speak at a school assembly? How do we know how many lives were changed by the realization that one has control over his or her body, that it can be made bigger, stronger, healthier?

We don't know. What is clear, though, is that Muscle Beach's greatest export wasn't photographs, movies, famous gyms, or gym equipment—it was people, before all else. It was the people from Muscle Beach who fanned out and influenced fitness around the world up to the present day.

"Actually," says Armand Tanny, "Muscle Beach was a mere postage stamp. It was a very exclusive club. It was a spot of numerous activities . . . it was novel. In itself . . . it never turned into a full-bore flame, except for the people who came out of it: my brother, Jack LaLanne, Harold Zinkin, Joe Gold. These guys went on to promote the business and promote the equipment.

"I think the core of the whole modern fitness movement was California," Tanny sums up. "It just spread from here, through these people, to everywhere else."